The Accidental

Health

Breakthrough

The Accidental Health Breakthrough: Implications for the Nation

---

Emilio Collar, Jr., PhD

Lisette Collar, RDMS

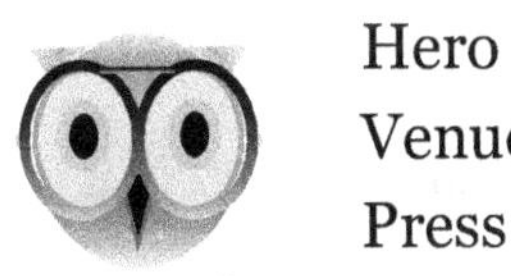

Hero
Venue
Press

www.herovenue.com

COPYRIGHT

First Printing, September 2021

Front-Page design by https://herovenue.com/

ISBN: 978-0-578-84953-9

Dedication

This book is dedicated to our devoted father, Emilio Collar, Sr., who coordinated the project and assisted us in doing research and conducting interviews with Cubans who lived in Cuba in the 1990s and now live in the United States. He made this work more relevant with his logic, insights, and historical knowledge.

And to the memory of our beloved mother, Juana Luisa, and our cherished uncle José Ángel Collar.

NUTRITIONAL HEALTH HONOR WALL

In recognition of the contributions of pioneers to the critical national debate on health, we acknowledge the thousands of researchers at the vanguard performing randomized trials at the cutting edge of investigations to uncover the facts.

Robert C. Atkins, MD
Edwin B. Astwood, MD
William Banting
Neal D. Barnard, MD
Claude Bernard, MD
Jeffrey S. Bland, PhD
Kelly D. Brownell, PhD
Will Bulsiewicz, MD
T. Colin Campbell, PhD
Thomas M. Campbell II, MD
Michael Eades, MD
Georgia Ede, MD
Eran Elinav, MD, PhD
Caldwell B. Esselstyn, Jr., MD
Joel Fuhrman, MD
Jason Fung, MD
Michael Greger MD
Jerome H. Grossman, MD
Jason Hwang, MD
Mark Hyman, MD
Chris A. Knobbe, MD
Ronald M. Krauss, MD
Chris Kresser, MD
Valter Longo, PhD
Robert H. Lustig, MD
Paul Mason, MD
Elmer V. McCollum, PhD
John McDougall, MD
Daphne Miller, MD
Marion Nestle, PhD
Dean Ornish, MD
Alfred W. Pennington, MD
David Perlmutter, MD
Stephen Phinney, MD, PhD
Michael Pollan
Pamela Popper, PhD, ND
Weston A. Price, DDS
Geoffrey Rose, MD
Eric M. Schlosser
Eran Segal, PhD
Catherine Shanahan, MD
Gerhard Spiteller, PhD
Gary Taubes
Nina Teicholz
Jeff Volek, PhD, RD
Terry Wahls, MD
Eric C. Westman, MD, MHS
John Yudkin, MD, PhD

CONTENTS

AT THE BEGINNING

It all began with a comprehensive physical examination, which I had put off for several years. I've always considered myself as relatively healthy, though a bit overweight. When I found out about my results, I was taken aback. I had high blood pressure and high cholesterol and was prediabetic. I was baffled as to how this could have occurred. Of course, my doctor prescribed various medications for me to take daily to alleviate the symptoms. The doctor assured me that the diseases would be manageable if I took the prescribed medicines for the rest of my life. He informed me that these are the most common chronic illnesses in the United States population. I suddenly felt like the poster person for contemporary chronic diseases. But, rather than relying just on my doctor's advice, I wanted to know how I acquired these conditions and what I could do about them. I decided to investigate the medical literature.

My medical condition was diagnosed as a "metabolic syndrome."[1] How about that? There was a fancy label for the condition! Chronic metabolic syndrome diseases are dangerous disorders. Some of the syndrome diseases are high blood pressure, elevated blood sugar (pre-diabetes), high cholesterol, and a large waist (obesity). Later in the book, we will discuss the syndrome and its diseases in more detail, and I will update you on my illness progress to share the lessons learned. Note: In this context, I'm referring only to me, Emilio, Jr. My sister, Lisette, is the one with a medical background and does not have the syndrome. On the contrary, she is exceptionally healthy and physically fit. She helped me research the subject and came up with the idea to write a book about our findings and conclusions. We devoted a significant amount of time to studying the medical literature. From here on out, we will be referring to both of us, so we'll use the pronoun "we."

Our initial goal was to compile the most up-to-date information on metabolic syndrome, how it emerged, and its impact on the population. During our research, we began to understand that the U.S. government dietary guidelines, although well-intentioned, had been a failed experiment for our nation's health. The nutritional guidelines have created the current health crisis (see Chapter 03). The United States has been on this dangerous trajectory for over 50 years. We began to outline this book based on what we had learned and our corresponding backgrounds. We started by asking ourselves some questions:

1. How did this unhealthy food environment develop in the United States?
2. Is there a solution to the U.S. health situation?
3. Can we identify a healthy food environment predicated on nutritional health principles?
4. Can a national nutritional strategy be developed and funded?

5. If not us, then who?

During our research, we came across an intriguing article on a health crisis in Cuba in the 1990s. The crisis started as a ripple in the cold North Atlantic Ocean and became a tsunami 7,000 miles away on an island in the warm Caribbean Sea. The ripple was the dissolution of the Soviet Union and the end of its aid to Cuba. The news hit the island like a tsunami and surged into an economic and health crisis. Cuba is 90 miles south of our shores, on the Florida straits. The island of Cuba is 1,250 kilometers long, with 11 million people primarily of Spanish and African descent. The research article was about a Cuban health crisis and postulated that some of the above-mentioned chronic disease incidences and mortality had decreased significantly. The paper was first published in the *American Journal of Epidemiology* in 2007 by a research team from Johns Hopkins School of Public Health in Baltimore.[2] An updated article, published in the *British Medical Journal* in 2013, was extensively quoted by the European press.[3]

We're not talking about Cuba's healthcare or political systems but rather the published research findings on the decline of chronic diseases in Cuba during the 1990s. The Cuban data was accessible to the researchers. The research article's key findings are (1) a 12-pound countrywide weight loss and the most significant results the decline in the incidence and mortality rates for (2) type 2 diabetes, (3) cardiovascular diseases, and (4) cancer.

Why do we think the findings of the Cuban study are relevant to health issues in the United States? The Cuban health crisis positively impacted chronic diseases associated with metabolic syndrome, the prevalent condition in the U.S. health crisis. The Cuban published research findings are consistent with our observations of chronic diseases in the U.S. population. The ***accidental health*** implications of Cuba's health crisis were extraordinary. The unexpected ***breakthrough*** was significant because it affected the entire country's population. Cuban health officials documented the health outcomes. What significance did these outcomes have for the United States? It demonstrated that the conditions that cause metabolic syndrome could be successfully addressed on a national scale and could be prevented and reversed relatively quickly. Moreover, during our investigation, we uncovered three additional factors in Cuba's health results that comprehensively explained the decline in chronic diseases. Chapter 2 will discuss the researchers' findings and the other variables in greater detail.

Based on the findings of the Cuban research, we decided to ask ourselves one more question;

6. Can some of the lessons learned from the Cuban health crisis be applied to the United States?

When feasible, we write in a conversational style, although the book may be more formal in some chapters due to the subject presented. We'll begin by looking at the current food landscape causing health problems in the United States. Our objective is to help the country by offering a proposal that will aid in reducing the country's most prevalent health problem, chronic metabolic syndrome diseases. We understand that those diseases are food-related.

To avoid detracting from the book's central theme, we've included appendices with extensive background information and helpful anchor points for readers who may seek additional knowledge.

So, we began to write this book.

Emilio Collar, Jr.

Lisette Collar

September 2021

CHAPTER 01.

THE WAY WE WERE: AN INTRODUCTION

We were reminiscing about our family and looking at photos of our parents and grandparents and their families and friends. At first, we didn't notice a striking feature on the pictures, but then it dawned on us: they were all thin. We're wondering if it was just our family. So we began searching the internet for older photographs of people from the 1950s and 1960s; those people were thin. It was unusual to find someone overweight, and it was usually an older person. When we compared those earlier photos to current ones, we were astounded by the physical differences. What happened to the people in the past 50 years?

We know that Americans today consume more unhealthy meals and are more sedentary than previous generations. However, it does not appear that this can explain the country's obesity problem. Obesity is evident, but also chronic disorders are increasing at significant annual rates. Other critical factors must be contributing to the obesity and chronic diseases in the population. As our research into those issues progressed, we realized that the United States is in the grip of a health catastrophe that is slowly killing us.

We the people... are sick!

Americans' life expectancy has been declining, attributed primarily to chronic metabolic syndrome diseases. Chronic metabolic syndrome diseases are dangerous conditions that many people are unaware of until it is too late. The American Heart Association defines metabolic syndrome as having 3 of the 5 following diseases: high blood pressure, high blood sugar level (pre-diabetes), low levels of good cholesterol (high-density lipids [HDLs]), high triglyceride levels, and a large waist (obesity) are the diseases (see Appendix D for more details).

In 1960, healthcare spending accounted for 5 percent of our gross domestic product (GDP). By 2020, it had grown fourfold to 20 percent of GDP, or more than $4 trillion, for the year.[4] We were a relatively healthy nation with predominantly normal-weight individuals until the 1970s. We have now become one of the most obese developed countries in the last 50 years. So, what went wrong? Our people's health, the national economy, and societal norms have all suffered because of this health situation.

The United States is in the midst of a self-inflicted health crisis resulting from a failed 50-year-long well-intentioned, but ill-advised dietary experiment. We began to realize that the United States government's dietary guidelines, while well-intended, had been a failed uncontrolled experiment for our country's health.[5] Government dietary guidelines are a strong suspect for the current health crisis. The crisis began after the United States Government issued the dietary guidelines to the nation. Since that time, it has progressed beyond a crisis to become a calamity. We use the term calamity literally to refer to a dire situation that causes long-term distress and suffering. For more than 50 years, the United States has been on this dangerous path. The health crisis appears to have been caused not by a scarcity of food but by an abundance of ultraprocessed and unhealthy food as the major contributing factor.[5-9] What are ultraprocessed foods? Highly processed or ultraprocessed foods have added ingredients such as sugar, salt, hydrogenated vegetable oils (trans fats), artificial colors, and preservatives. Also, additives and emulsifiers such as artificial flavors, refined sugars, added salt, stabilizers, and others are included. They have eye-catching packaging, and bold health label claims. They are the most profitable segment of Big Food companies' portfolios.[10]

There is little doubt that Americans today eat more calories from ultraprocessed foods and are more sedentary than Americans 50 years ago, from children to adults.[11] Is it our way of life that's getting us sick, or is it what we eat, or both? We are obese compared with our parents and grandparents. That is a fact. But what about other reasons? Is it possible that the food we eat is different? What about the fast foods and convenience foods we consume? Do we consume too much food during the day? Who is responsible for keeping people healthy? In the following chapters, we'll address those concerns.

Asking the Important Questions

In the United States, a patchwork of conflicting answers will not provide a complete solution to a complex health problem. We're attempting to postulate a proposal for a solution to the leading health issue. We present a mental roadmap with which you may follow our rationale using the tried-and-true questions of why, what, who, where, how, and when.

Why? **Why are we sick?** We have a food technology culture that embraces the maxim that **industrialized human-made food can be superior to natural food.** Nutritionist scientists who work for food companies believe that enriching industrialized processed food can supply the essential nutrients for human health. Nutritionism is a term coined by Michael Pollan to describe this type of dietary orthodoxy. Dr. Robert Lustig calls industrialized food the commoditization of the foods we eat.[6, 8, 9] Despite the food scientist's best efforts, high processed or ultraprocessed food is not nutritional and causes metabolic syndrome in the population.

What? **What is making us sick?** Chronic diseases are nutritional in nature and can be traced back to **ultraprocessed foods with added sugar and seed or grain (vegetable) oils.** We know it as the Western diet. The NOVA classification categorizes food products depending on their degree of processing, and it includes ultraprocessed foods as one of the four groups. Food industrialization is a global phenomenon; the same chronic diseases found in America begin to appear in other nations when those nations adopt the Western diet.[12] Slow-acting toxic substances in the processed foods we eat progressively make us sick and eventually kill us prematurely.[13]

Who? Who is making us sick? Food companies, U.S. government agencies, and some medical organizations have been complicit in promoting the Western diet of high-carbohydrate/low-fat processed foods containing sugars and seed or grain (vegetable) oils as a healthy diet. As a result, we are experiencing the worst health crisis in the history of our country.[5] As the Western diet becomes more popular in countries outside of the United States, the same diseases arise in those countries.

Where? Where are we eating this food? In the United States, ultraprocessed foods have become ubiquitous. **From supermarkets to fast-food outlets to restaurant chains and neighborhood restaurants, these foods are readily available**. This type of food accounts for *60 percent* of our daily calorie intake. The percentage is higher in low-income and minority communities because these foods are inexpensive. Processed food is also the most profitable food commodity for food manufacturers, and it is extensively advertised and sold worldwide.[14]

How? **How do we turn this health calamity around?** Part of the solution to this catastrophe can be found in the lessons learned from Cuba's 1990s health crisis (see Chapter 02 for details). Some of the Cuban lessons may be applicable in the United States.[2] We may use this knowledge to propose **healthy living solutions** to address the U.S. health crisis. Traditional healthcare does not attempt to prevent this health disaster. Our healthcare system is a mechanism for diagnosing and treating illnesses. Pharmaceutical companies' medications, which the Food and Drug Administration (FDA) has approved, only treat the symptoms of chronic diseases, not the underlying causes. There are no financial incentives for the medical or pharmaceutical industries to implement a nutritional approach to prevent disease.[13]

When? **When can we expect an improvement in our national health?** It will be up to us, the citizens of this country, to decide. To solve the current health crisis, we propose a national nutritional health strategy based on healthy foods. Assume we can gain U.S. Congressional support and public approval to begin living a healthy lifestyle. In that instance, **after the first year of implementation**, positive health outcomes will start to emerge. Within 5 years of its health crisis, Cuba achieved a significant reversal of metabolic syndrome disorders. There is no reason why we shouldn't be able to do just as well.[3]

If Not Us, Then Who?

Despite their good intentions, the U.S. government's dietary guidelines supported by medical organizations have failed to improve our country's health. Every American is affected by the present health crisis.[5] It has had an impact on worker productivity as well as the economic wealth of our society. We've studied and reviewed many band-aid remedies proposed to stop the bleeding of a hemorrhaging patient to use a medical metaphor.

We asked ourselves the question: what are we attempting to achieve with this book? We investigated the Cuban health crisis and learned about the burdens it imposed as well as the ones it alleviated. If we could use what we've learned, we might provide another path in the United States to help improve people's health. We couldn't just sit on the sidelines and claim that the country has a health problem; we needed to go beyond simple statements. Perhaps, we could contribute to improving the health situation in the U.S. We decided to consolidate a patchwork of viable solutions into a cohesive plan to address the United States health calamity.

This book will not rehash medical studies or historical conclusions; many people knowledgeable on the issue have already done so in recent years. Some of their books and articles are cited in the References section of this book. Many facets of the health problem have been identified so far by researchers and several brilliant writers. We'll use everything we've learned so far to develop a workable and acceptable solution to our nation's health crisis.

We realized that our country's self-inflicted tragedy might be best addressed at the national level as we read about the Cuban crisis. It can, however, also be addressed on an individual basis, but it will take a lot longer. A countrywide solution requires a concerted effort, yet there has been and continues to be none. The medical system and pharmaceutical businesses have no financial incentive to provide a healthy food solution. There is no national organization dedicated to improving people's health. As a result, the health catastrophe continues unabated.

To prevent the situation from worsening further, we need a practical solution that addresses the core causes of the health disaster. Our investigation into the Cuban health crisis recognized that metabolic syndrome could be reversed in a few short years if the solution was applied nationwide. We offer practical proposals for reversing the calamity on a personal and national level.

The issues will be laid out in the book as we see them. We are convinced that, first and foremost, people's health should be prioritized. We need to provide the people suffering a way out of their predicament. The solution will also allow the government, medical institutions, and enterprises that caused the problem to help improve the citizens' and shareholders' health.

We must face the harsh reality that those institutions have failed the country, and they now bear the responsibility of making things right. This tragedy has affected us all. If people's health is not a top concern for any organization in the country, it is time to establish a nonprofit organization dedicated solely to that goal. We are going to propose an individual and national strategy for healthy living in the public forum. We feel that a partial or tentative solution will simply push our country closer to the brink. We'll briefly look into the Cuban health crisis in the next section to understand how it may relate to the health challenges in the United States and explore that crisis in more detail in Chapter 2.

If not us, then who? Now we know. **The answer is us.**

Notable Events of 1990s Cuba

Cubans (mostly of Spanish and African descent) are remarkable people who, since colonial times, have struggled for independence and freedom. They were unintentionally caught up in a significant historical event at the end of the 20th century: the Soviet Union's breakdown in 1989 culminated in its total dissolution in 1991.[15] The Soviets provided financial aid to Cuba since 1961, but when the Soviet bloc disintegrated, the aid abruptly ceased in

1990, resulting in an economic and health crisis in the 1990s. The health improvements that occurred in Cuba throughout that decade are of great importance to us as a country today.

Chapter 2 will look at the Cuban health crisis and its consequences and how it relates to current metabolic syndrome research. The research relationship could help us explain the Cuban health implications and how they relate to the US health situation. We want to learn from it and see if the lessons can be applied in the United States. The word "accidental" is included in the book title because the phenomenon under investigation occurred unpredictably and had unexpected consequences. Cuba's health crisis was unusual for a country at peace. It has enabled us to understand a few critical variables affecting the health of a nation of 11-million people. As mentioned earlier, health officials in Cuba documented the health results in their population.

The United States Health Environment

Researching the causes of the metabolic syndrome took us a couple of years. We grew discouraged during our research into the medical literature. We realized that our healthcare system was not designed to cure chronic diseases but was set up to treat and manage symptoms.[16, 17] Cure differs from treatment in that cure usually refers to a complete recovery from an illness. On the other hand, treatment refers to the processes that lead to improving health through disease management. Physicians frequently refer to chronic diseases as "manageable diseases."

The pharmaceutical business and the medical establishment in the United States are focused on treating ailments.[17] Treatments for high blood pressure, obesity, diabetes, heart disease, cancer, pain, and other chronic conditions have made tremendous progress and profits for those institutions. They should be commended for the medical and pharmaceutical remedies they have developed to manage those ailments, but they have not cured them. For healthcare treatment, the free market has functioned successfully; the incentives and rewards are clear.

When we say that the term *metabolic syndrome* defines modern chronic diseases, we mean it; these diseases are modern. They're also known as diseases of modern civilization.[18] The World Health Organization (WHO) calls them non-communicable diseases.[13] In the 19th century, these diseases were almost unknown. In the second half of the 20th century, they began to appear in large numbers among the population. The diseases began by food companies accelerating the production of ultraprocessed foods with high carbs in collaboration with the U.S. Government. If this tendency continues, our healthcare system will be insolvent by 2026, resulting in healthcare rationing.[6, 19] It's not always a bad thing to spend more on healthcare, especially if it results in better health outcomes. In the United States, however, this is not the case. Despite higher healthcare spending, the United States lags behind other countries in standard health metrics.[4]

These metabolic syndrome diseases account for more than 75 percent of current U.S. healthcare spending, and the number is rising, posing a financial and societal threat to our nation.

The Evolving Status of Twenty-First Century Nutritional Health

With a better understanding of nutrition, the general public's perceptions of a healthy diet are evolving. A new generation of physicians and researchers is more pragmatic than previous generations. They base the national debate on food on scientific facts rather than outdated dogmas, using biochemistry and randomized research.[9] They also realize that there is no one-size-fits-all diet for the entire population. Future healthy diets must be tailored based on age, gender, and underlying health issues, at the very least. According to our findings, people are skeptical about governmental dietary guidelines, certified dietitians, and professional medical associations that support the guidelines. In the worst situations, people do not have confidence in those organizations. Despite randomized controlled trials revealing the harmful consequences of their low-fat, high-carbohydrate diet on the nation's population, those officials refuse to consider changing their past policies. The United States Department of Agriculture's (USDA) MyPlate dietary guidelines are just the latest incarnation of the same old diet with its perplexing guidelines.[5]

The health crisis would be considered a national security concern if our food were a military issue. But wait, it is a military issue when almost one-quarter of the young people applying to the military are rejected due to metabolic syndrome. It is an insidious threat that has a negative impact on citizens' productivity. A considerable amount of the (GDP) is spent on health-related issues.[20-23] By lowering labor productivity, health issues jeopardize the nation's long-term viability. We cannot keep ignoring this national issue.

Leading with Research: An Emergent Proposal

We wondered if Cuba's unintentional health results could be replicated in the United States without the food scarcity crisis that triggered them in Cuba. But then, we must recognize that our country is in the midst of a health crisis. It is not a lack-of-food crisis, as it was in Cuba, but rather a crisis caused by an abundance of ultraprocessed unhealthy food. This abundance is more than a source of concern; it is a calamity! We know how to deal with an abundance of food. We gain weight. We also know how to deal with food scarcity; it's been a part of human life for millennia, and our metabolism has evolved to manage it.[24] The research on the Cuban health crisis validates this fact.

The food technology that produces ultraprocessed food and its abundance is the leading cause of metabolic syndrome diseases among Americans and most peoples of the world.[14] The effects of these foods are particularly noticeable among low-income and minority groups, as the foods are inexpensive and hence consumed in large quantities by those demographic groups. These groups have also had some of the highest rates of coronavirus.[25] Poor-quality (ultraprocessed) food did not help; it created their underlying chronic illnesses, and their compromised immune systems could not fight the coronavirus. The virus's mortality rates in low-income and minority groups back up this suspicion.[26, 27]

Our research has resulted in a possible strategy for addressing health challenges in the United States. It indicated that we should look into processed food technology, the companies that make processed foods, and the government regulations that support it.

The following factors were considered:

- The Western diet, which includes ultraprocessed convenience foods as a significant component
- The United States government's dietary recommendations for the general population and the causes of obesity
- Cuba's health crisis and its implications to the United States
- The adverse effects of a sedentary lifestyle
- Diseases associated with metabolic syndrome and its causes
- Lack of nutritional knowledge in the general public

- The existing treatment-oriented healthcare system
- Factors that contribute to a healthy lifestyle

We realized that all of these issues are closely intertwined. Identifying the connections between those topics could help us better understand the problem.

A National Perspective: Focus on Health

The COVID-19 pandemic has exposed the shortcomings in our existing healthcare system, particularly those that affect low-income workers and minorities.[26] Our current healthcare system, a marvel of modern medicine, is mainly successful in treating and managing chronic diseases and other disorders. It is beneficial to most middle-class workers and persons over the age of 65. Compared to other free-market countries, the United States spends more than twice as much per capita on healthcare as other industrialized countries. There are 39 countries with longer life expectancies than the United States, despite spending less on healthcare per capita than the U.S.[28]

The Affordable Care Act (ACA) failed to address the most important aspects of optimal health: nutrition and lifestyle. **You cannot fix people's health until you fix their diet.**[29] The ACA makes no provisions for chronic disease prevention; it solely covers their treatment.[30]. The ACA intended to lower healthcare costs by promoting preventative medicine, but no allowances were made for it in the bill. Ezekiel J. Emanuel was aware of this, and he penned a magazine article expressing his desire to die at the age of 75.[31] Was it possible that the only way the ACA could lower healthcare expenses was for Americans to die prematurely?

Why was the ACA's approach to preventative care unworkable?

- The ACA did not include any preventative medicine or healthy living provisions, such as those for good nutrition and physical activity.
- Preventive medicine cannot be implemented using the existing healthcare system.
- The current U.S. healthcare is a fragmented system of physicians, specialized treatment, and hospitals designed to treat illness.
- Furthermore, the preventative approach can lower the earnings of the medical profession and pharmaceutical firms.
- Consequently, most of them would oppose a preventative approach surreptitiously.

When discussing the government's dietary guidelines, we should use the term *legacy*. No matter how well-intentioned, regrettably, the preceding generation of Americans has left us with an unhealthy legacy of their making.[5, 32] We hope, however, that future generations will be able to successfully reverse that harmful tendency, create healthier solutions for our country, and leave a healthy American legacy for future generations. The current generation must recognize that our country is steadily falling into a food swamp and must move onto a natural solid ground before drowning.

We Are a Nation of Innovators, Entrepreneurs, and Doers

Since its inception, our country has been a nation of entrepreneurs, always coming up with new ideas and successfully reimagining and enhancing previous ones. Initially referred to as a paradigm shift, the process is now referred to as a disruption in today's millennial parlance. As a nation, we can develop an effective nutritional health strategy. First and foremost, personalized healthy nutrition should be emphasized, with natural food taking precedence over other lifestyle aspects and physical activity as an essential component of good health.

We cringed whenever we saw an entrepreneur food product on the Shark Tank TV show (our favorite) prepared with unhealthy and harmful ingredients (refined white flour, sugar, salt, vegetable oils, and long shelf-life emulsifiers) or an unhealthy new fast-food outlet. Worse, investors who should know better outbid themselves to bring the dangerous product or fast-food restaurant to market. They should serve as a national model of ethical investors aiding entrepreneurs in introducing healthy food options to the market to assist the country in overcoming our health crisis. TV producers should be more health-conscious and avoid promoting unhealthy entrepreneurial food products on their Shark Tank television show.

We need to level the playing field for the typical consumer versus the food giants' dominating public advertising. The only way to fight the food industry's advertising juggernaut is with a focused public education advertising campaign that explains the benefits of consuming healthy natural food or minimally processed food versus ultraprocessed food. The approach should be implemented on a national basis and widely publicized. This strategy will assist in reducing our present healthcare expenditures without interfering with treatment technologies for people who are or will become ill.

Chronic Metabolic Syndrome Diseases

Appendix D contains a description of some of the previously mentioned chronic illnesses. We debated whether to include this appendix as our book progressed. Despite this, we feel that metabolic syndrome should be made more widely known. Consumers must understand the chronic metabolic syndrome disorders that underpin the syndrome and their most significant complication, type 2 diabetes. As a result, Appendix D is a valuable resource for readers seeking a basic understanding of these heinous diseases.

The Global Food Environment

The Western diet has evolved into the primary driver of chronic diseases worldwide, described as non-communicable diseases by the World Health Organization. The following chapters present a historical overview of the Western diet and food technology progress during the previous 50 years. The general public is unaware of the complete and pervasive influence of the food industry in today's global food environment and culture. Food corporations wield unprecedented power over the global food supply, unchallenged by any government. We have modified the adage; power corrupts, and when it is global, it corrupts even the politicians elected to limit the power of those corporations.

The following chapters...

- You've already read the first chapter, which provides an overview of the United States' uncontrollable health experiment.
- Chapter 02 will provide an overview of how the Cuban health crisis may bear lessons for the United States after more than 50 years of the most ill-advised health experiment in our country's history.
- Chapter 03 will examine how we got into this health crisis and the main characters in this real-life drama. It will all revolve around how food corporations have altered our

food over time, making it more processed, harmful, and convenient. It has given food companies greater control over the food supply chain while increasing their political clout in Congress.

- In Chapters 04 to 07, we'll explore the connection between natural (real) food and health, as well as how it might aid in the cure of diseases. We'll examine long-forgotten dietary habits as well as ones that improve health and prevent disease.
- Chapter 08 will assess COVID-19's impact on our country and some lessons for the future.
- In Chapter 09, we will describe principles of natural nutrition that you can implement as an individual to improve your health and quality of life.
- Chapter 10 will discuss the need for a public, non-profit organization to educate the public about nutrition and the chemicals in our food supply without being influenced by the food industry.
- Chapter 11 will put forward a national nutritional strategy and campaign to lessen the health crisis by educating the public on the proper foods to eat and being physically active to improve their quality of life.
- Chapter 12 will present a new health policy and economic concept to help fund the nation's nutritional strategy.

- In Chapter 13, the cost and savings considerations associated with metabolic syndrome diseases will be discussed.

We sincerely hope you enjoy this book and support its recommendations. First and foremost, we must address our country's health calamity. A national health crisis in another country under difficult and unexpected circumstances could assist us in that endeavor. Understanding those variables can contribute to enhancing our country's health. We can improve people's lives by leveraging and adapting existing technologies in our country, training physicians and nutritionists in biochemistry, launching a public awareness campaign about the dangers of processed foods, and educating the public about natural foods and physical activity. Our proposal has the potential to pave the way for a new health paradigm in the United States.

In Appendix A, we describe in detail the events that led to the health crisis in Cuba. It provides health lessons that can apply to the global community.

§ § §

CHAPTER 02.

NINETY MILES AWAY FROM A MAJOR HEALTH CRISIS

A health catastrophe 90 miles south of our shores, in the Florida Straits, may have suggested an answer to America's health crisis. The disaster began in 1989 when the Cuban economy began to crumble due to the Soviet Union's disintegration. Because much of Cuba's trade was with the USSR and its Soviet republics, global commerce dropped by roughly 80% during that time. Cuba's GDP fell by 40 to 50 percent during that timeframe. The government adopted certain aspects of capitalism to save its communist revolution. Cuba permitted foreign investment in resort hotels to accommodate international tourists. It leased farm property to private farmers since the confiscation of all farmland in 1961 and allowed private farmer's markets. It legalized the use of U.S. dollars and self-employment in new small private enterprises such as restaurants, coffee shops, and pastry stores.

In addition to the international political forces that precipitated the crisis, it was aggravated by Cuba's domestic economic policies. The Cuban economy, like that of most socialist regimes, is managed through central planning. Its 5-year plan could not adapt to the new economic reality, causing the economy to deteriorate further. The Cuban government's economic planning throughout the years had not produced enough food to feed its people. The planned economy had been a colossal failure.[28]

Although the communist bloc nations of the former Soviet Union were able to adopt free-market policies and transform their economies, Cuba could not do so. The Cuban Communist Party is made up of dogmatic Marxist/Leninist linear thinkers who are incapable of straying from the fundamentals of a failed ideology. Although the communist party accepted free market features during the severe economic crisis to save its communist revolution, it began to reverse such policies in the early 2000s as its economy recovered. Anyone who observes the realities of life in Cuba will see the absurd consequences of obsessively focusing on a social ideology and a planned economy.

Since taking power in 1959, Cuba's communist government has made no effort to modernize, develop, or invest in new industries. The Soviet Union's substantial financial assistance ($65 billion) has been squandered on fomenting communist uprisings in Africa and Latin America. To top it all off, Cuba has maintained a significant annual budget deficit in its international trade since the revolution. The communist ideology of Cuba is incompatible with modern economic concepts. Cubans follow the failed economic communist models of Joseph Stalin and Mao Zedong rather than Deng Xiaoping's free-market model. China and Vietnam are communist nations that have largely abandoned the notion of a planned economy in favor of free-market principles, resulting in thriving economies and lifting its people from poverty. Due to the narrow ideological emphasis, domestic actions in Cuba have been insufficient in alleviating the country's economic and health difficulties throughout the crisis.

The health crisis had an accidental health benefit, however. Many Cubans lost a significant amount of weight, and more importantly, the incidence and mortality rates of diabetes, heart disease, and cancer were also significantly reduced. The unexpected breakthrough was significant because it included the entire nation's population. How might that benefit us in the United States? The Cuban health crisis was the first Western nation to demonstrate that these chronic diseases could be successfully reversed at a national level relatively quickly.

Medical researchers saw the Cuban health crisis as a great opportunity. It was a situation caused by political events in a time of peace, not by war or natural catastrophe. News accounts from that period reported on and analyzed Cuba's economic situation (see Appendix A for more details. The *American Journal of Epidemiology* published an article in 2007 that explored this period in Cuba from a health perspective; it is the only credible academic research paper we've found that discussed the health crisis.[2] An article with updated research appeared in the *British Medical Journal* in April 2013. The study's objective was to evaluate the population-wide weight loss and the incidence and mortality rates of diabetes and mortality trends in cardiovascular disease and cancer in Cuba over a 30-year interval.[3] There were news reports about food scarcity during that decade, but they lacked any health data to analyze the effects on the population.

Summary of Research Findings

Due to food scarcity, the loss of weight in the general population of Cuba was significant. The result was not an anecdotal account in a diet book about some individuals losing weight; it was, instead, a factual report on the people of an entire nation. The significance of weight loss by itself is not that important. Still, it gave us empirical (derived from experience or observation) data showing that specific dietary conditions can improve a nation's health. The most important findings of the research are the chronic metabolic syndrome disease results.[3] The incidences and mortality reduction of type 2 diabetes, cardiovascular diseases, and cancer have extraordinary ramifications for America's health calamity.

Here is a summary of the Cuban results:[2, 3]

- In the 1990s, Cuban people had an average weight decline of 12 pounds (5.5 kilograms). It was primarily due to the scarcity of food during that period. Cubans did not tend to be obese; on the contrary, most of the population was normal-weight.
- The weight loss was attributed to a low caloric intake and high caloric expenditure. Because of a lack of fuel oil,

transportation was limited or non-existent, and Cubans had to bike or walk from place to place. The theory behind the research seemed to be that the calories-in, calories-out process of weight loss had occurred. However, from recent randomized trials, we know that that theory is flawed. Calories were not the leading cause of weight loss but only one factor (see below, Additional Revealing Factors).

- The incidence and mortality rates from diabetes were cut by 50 percent during that period.
- The mortality rate of cardiovascular disease was reduced by 33% during that period.
- The mortality rate of cancer was reduced by 2.4 percent during that period.

The last three bullets above should be of critical importance to the United States. We will explore those factors in more detail. You should know that food in Cuba has always been scarce, but it was exceedingly scarce in the first half of the 1990s. The revolutionary government had established food rationing 30 years earlier. Each person could buy fixed quantities of food at certain times of the month based on family size and availability at government grocery stores. The government distributed food to the stores, and each Cuban was required to use a *libreta de abastecimiento* (grocery food booklet) to buy the food. Food could also be bought on the black market, which has been pervasive in Cuba for many years.

Additional Revealing Factors

Cubans are remarkable people, and we do not want to minimize their suffering during that decade or belittle some of their illnesses, such as neuropathy, dysfunction of one or more nerves caused by vitamin deficiency due to a lack of sufficient nutrients.[33] We hope that the health results of their ordeal can be a silver lining to help us in the United States understand our health calamity and apply some Cuban health variables. The importance of the research is not that it revealed the average amount of weight loss in the national population of Cuba. The majority of the people in Cuba in the 1990s were already of what we in the United States call normal weight. Their loss of weight resulted from the scarcity of food available to them. The Cubans' weight-loss implications may be exciting for the current U.S. population, about half of whom are overweight.

The fascinating and essential facts found in the Cuban research are the 50-percent reduction in the incidence and mortality rates of type 2 diabetes, the 33-percent reduction in cardiovascular mortality rates, and the 2.4-percent reduction in cancer mortality rates during that period. Those variables are the critical findings of the research, and they have led us to ask some obvious questions: What factors influenced those results? What lessons can we learn from that experience? The Cubans' weight loss was one factor in reversing their chronic diseases, but it was not the only factor, so what were the others? We are attempting to understand and connect it to current health research in the United States.

We uncovered three additional revealing factors not considered in the original research that comprehensively explained the Cuban health results. We discovered these interesting factors by interviewing Cubans who lived through that period in Cuba and currently reside in the United States.

1. **It was the food.** Cubans ate a natural (real) food diet free of ultraprocessed foods, refined grains, seed oils, refined sugar, and sugary drinks during the crisis. They could not purchase processed foods and refined grains from overseas due to a lack of foreign currency. They also lack fuel oil for electrical power plants and transportation of goods and services. Even sugar cane was in short supply. As a result of the crisis, Cuba's food environment shifted from a Western diet to a natural organic diet.
2. **It was the lack of food at certain times.** Some days during the month, there was no food to eat. As a result, Cubans inadvertently practiced *intermittent fasting* at certain times of the month because there was not enough food available until the day they could get it at government groceries on their rationing schedule.
3. **It was the timing for eating.** Cubans only ate two or three times a day. They needed to conserve food. There was no food for snacking. There were many days in the month when no breakfast was available, and people ate only two meals or one meal a day to preserve food. We call that form of eating *time-*

restricted feeding, and it is a variation of intermittent fasting. But, again, it did not happen by design but due to the economic conditions.

The study attributed the positive weight loss in Cuba to energy (calorie) reduction and energy (calorie) expenditure. We now know that the assumption about caloric reduction is flawed. Research in the last few years has validated that as a person reduces caloric intake, the body lowers the caloric expenditure to match the intake. For example, if a person eats 2,500 calories a day and then drops the intake to 1,800 calories, the calorie expenditure is also reduced to 1,800 calories. Hormones and metabolic rates regulate our bodies.[24, 34] Lower calorie intake only leads to hunger.[8]

Due to the restrictive premise of their calories-in, calories-out hypothesis during that period, the researchers did not consider the Cuban diet an essential question; possibly, there was no data available. However, proper natural nutrition is a more critical factor than caloric intake in losing weight and reducing type 2 diabetes and obesity [1].

Even though the food was scarce, most of the food that **Cubans ate was natural food**. Overseas permaculturists, who study

---

[1] Note that the Cuban people, by Western standards, were not overweight. Although we have obese people with metabolic syndrome in the United States, we have a higher number of normal-weight people with the syndrome (see Appendix D). Normal-weight people in the United States weigh about the same as the average Cuban did before the 1990s crisis. U.S. researchers have found that normal-weight people in the United States who have metabolic syndrome tend to rely heavily on the Western diet of ultraprocessed convenience foods and sugary drinks.[32]

human habits and food production systems, arrived in Cuba at the time and taught their techniques to locals, who soon implemented them in fields, raised beds, and urban plots across the nation. Organic agriculture was instituted after a mandate by the government because the government could not afford chemical fertilizers. To supplement the foods that were hard to produce, the government provided vegetable seeds, predominantly for green vegetables, that were easy to grow so that individuals might start their own vegetable gardens.

During the health crisis, the Cuban government allowed private organic farming on farms and organic urban farming on any empty plot of land in the cities (see Appendix A). Cubans had no choice but to eat a rationed organic green vegetable diet. We assert that the researchers neglected to include the people's diet as a variable in their analysis. Although they did not have it as a variable in their research, they indirectly broached the subject in their paper.[3]

Cubans also occasionally ate meats and poultry (pork and chicken mostly; it is a crime to kill a bull or cow because it is needed for milk) and wild-caught fish available on the black market. The Cuban people with families overseas received money from them to buy food on the black market. (Be aware that more than 1 million people, or about 10% of the population, had fled the island in the 30 years prior to the crisis.) The pork and chicken the Cubans ate were pasture-raised by local farmers since no animal feeds were available, and local fishers caught wild fish. There was no refrigeration or means of transporting the fish, but that was not much of a problem because Cuba is a long narrow island (1,250 kilometers) surrounded by bountiful seas. Most of the fish caught were eaten locally. Many Cubans had no access to dollars and no way of buying food on the black market. They suffered the most because the food distributed by the government was not very abundant. The decline in food availability was associated with a neuropathy outbreak in the adult population in the mid-1990s.[2, 28]

Cubans had no choice but to eat natural (real) foods. During the first half of the 1990s, processed foods of any kind were nonexistent. They could not be imported because of government-imposed import restrictions (due to the lack of foreign currency), and they could not be manufactured (due to a lack of electricity) or transported (due to a lack of fuel oil) in Cuba. The absence of unhealthy, industrialized processed foods and sugary beverages was another reason type 2 diabetes and heart disease rates fell, and weight loss became common.

The second significant factor that was not studied by the researchers but had a substantial impact on the Cuban population's positive health results was the **inadvertent practice of intermittent fasting.** Cubans did not intend to fast; they had to fast because of their circumstances. Fasting initiates specific hormonal adaptations (see Chapter 7). Fasting allows insulin levels to drop significantly, preventing insulin resistance, which leads to type 2 diabetes, and maintaining a high metabolic rate.[24] Fasting helps burn fat stored in the body's cells, reducing glucose levels, triggering autophagy, and causing weight loss (see Appendix D).

Fasting also lowers insulin resistance and reverses diabetes in a short time.[35, 36] According to Dr. Jason Fung, fasting provides beneficial hormonal changes.[37] Fasting is a powerful tool for reducing and reversing type 2 diabetes. Fasting and its benefits are the most likely reasons for Cuba's remarkable reduction in type 2 diabetes. Diabetes is the dominant disease in metabolic syndrome.

The third revealing factor was the inadvertent practice of time-restricted feeding. Once again, Cubans were not trying to restrict their feeding time but were forced to do so by their prevailing circumstances. Time-restricted feeding involves eating only for a certain number of hours each day. By skipping a meal, usually breakfast, one can fast for 16 hours and then have 8 nonfasting hours (i.e., have lunch and dinner during those 8 hours). This schedule is based on the circadian rhythms, which control every hormone. Time-restricted feeding appears to give the body time to repair itself.[38, 39] Furthermore, Cubans did not snack between meals because snacks were not available.

The following research supports the previously uncovered, revealing factors correlated with the health improvements in the Cuban population. First, a study by Dr. Caldwell Esselstyn, Jr., in *Prevent and Reverse Heart Disease*[17] discusses the decline in heart disease and deaths associated with a plant-based diet that excludes vegetable oils, which were not available in Cuba. Second, Dr. Jason Fung's research in *The Obesity Code,*[24] *The Diabetes Code*[37] and *The Cancer Code*[40] explains how intermittent fasting can lead to weight loss, a decline in the incidence of diabetes, and other health benefits. Third, a study by Dr. Robert Lustig in *Fat Chance*[6] also describes the positive impact of eliminating ultraprocessed fast foods and refined sugar on weight loss and metabolic syndrome diseases. The health factors identified by those authors' research were present during the health crisis in Cuba.

The Cuban Experience: Nutritional Factors

The following empirical factors played a significant role in Cuba's national health results based on research papers, news sources, and interviews with Cubans who lived through that period in Cuba and currently live in the United States.

1. There was a lack of ultraprocessed foods, refined grains, seed and grain (vegetable) oils, refined sugar, and sugary beverages.
2. A typical diet was composed of organic green vegetables, rice, and dry legumes (primarily black beans).
3. Occasionally, pasture-raised chicken and pork and locally caught wild fish were available for purchase or on the black market.
4. There was no snacking between meals because snacks were not available.
5. One or two meals a day were the norm, and coffee was drunk at breakfast if it was available.

6. Intermittent fasting and time-restricted feeding were inadvertently practiced at times during the month.
7. A regiment of daily physical activity of riding a bicycle or walking to work or the grocery store was normal.
8. According to our Cuban sources, people drank a lot of water during the day because they were hungry most of the time. We have not independently verified this factor, although it makes sense given Cuba's humid and hot climate. Because there was no power to provide air conditioning, a person would need to drink a lot of water to stay hydrated.

As you can see from the list above, Cubans mostly ate organic vegetables without industrialized processed fast foods, added chemicals, and refined food products. They also ate saturated fats from pasture-raised poultry and pork, as well as omega-3 fats from fish. They ate very few, if any, omega-6 fats (i.e., no seed or grain oils). They ate no snacks between meals. They engaged in intermittent fasting and time-restricted feeding at times during the month and drank a lot of water during the day. A significant level of daily physical activity accompanied this diet. When food is scarce and people are hungry, it is difficult to give a diet a name, but whatever food was available was healthy and natural (real) and resulted in unexpected health outcomes.

Despite the hardships, the Cuban people have achieved something that no other Western country has accomplished. In just 5 years, they lost weight and, more significantly, lowered the incidence and mortality rates of chronic metabolic syndrome disorders such as type 2 diabetes, cardiovascular diseases, and cancer. Furthermore, their experience has demonstrated that these disorders could be treated across the country using a natural (real) food diet of green vegetables, meat, fish, physical activity, and time-restricted feeding.

Subsequently, as part of a national effort to make and keep people healthy, we will discuss how we may adapt some of the health factors. To do this, we will outline and propose a nutritional health strategy. But first, we must understand the main reasons and the evolution of our self-inflicted health crisis in the United States. The Cuban experience, although unfortunate, proves a 2,500 years old healthy truth postulated by Hippocrates of Kos, the father of medicine, "Let thy food be your medicine, and medicine be thy food."

§ § §

Chapter 03.

A Real-Life Health Mystery: Who's the Villain?

What captures our attention in mystery novels or films is unraveling the mystery and figuring out who the villain is in the drama. We look for clues and put them together to identify the bad guys while we read or watch a film. The mystery is exposed, and the villain is recognized after the story comes to an end. We have a true mystery in our life, much like in novels or films. The risk of diabetes, obesity, cardiovascular disease, cancer, dementia, joint pain, and other chronic diseases is significantly higher than before the 1950s. Why?

We want to find the villains of this health disaster. Numerous books and research articles on the issue have been published in recent years, identifying pieces of the jigsaw puzzle. As a result, we will focus on the most critical aspects of the research and health crisis. For more details, please check the publications listed in the References.

First Suspect: Industrialized Unhealthy Foods

We need to find some leads on the suspects. Because obesity is increasing dramatically worldwide, let's start with food. Japan's traditional diet includes white rice (carbohydrates), fish (proteins), soybeans (proteins and fiber), and vegetables (nutrients and fiber).[41] This diet can be classified as a low-fat diet. The quantities are small, and meals are typically served three times a day. People who follow this diet are not obese and do not suffer from chronic metabolic illnesses. Something changed in Japan in the 1980s: the introduction of Western fast-food outlets serving ultraprocessed foods.

Today, the island of Okinawa, where people used to live to be 100 years old, has the highest obesity rate of any Japanese district.[42] Obesity affected 20 percent of the Japanese population in 2012, a threefold increase since the 1960s; even children are becoming obese.[43] The prevalence of metabolic syndrome is now increasing in the population.[14] This is also the case in other Asian countries, including China, where ultraprocessed fast foods have been introduced.[44, 45] Therefore, any ultraprocessed fast food is a strong suspect.

Following World War II, ultraprocessed foods began to emerge on grocery store shelves in greater numbers. They were promoted as being both convenient and nutritious for a healthy country. Food, according to Dr. Robert Lustig, has evolved from a necessity to a commercial commodity. As a result, it has been modified in the last

50 years to be an addictive substance. We are getting sick because the existing food environment generated by the processed food industry does not match the biochemical nature of humans.[8, 46, 47]

We Americans are marveled and obsessed with technology and all things related to it. While valid in many aspects of our lives, the truism does not apply to food. We have enthusiastically embraced industrialized ultraprocessed meals as the most modern and easy meals to consume. Food industry nutritionists do not understand how natural food nutrients and chemicals interact in an edible plant or how removing some of them, such as the nutrients in refined white flour, affects human health. They can recognize vitamins and minerals and break down the meal into proteins, carbs, lipids (fats), and fibers. They are, however, perplexed as to how it all interacts with and affects the human body. It's similar to cracking an egg, extracting most of the yolk and white, enriching it with synthetic nutrients, and adding chemicals for flavors, sugar to make it sweet, and preservatives. Finally, you reassemble the egg, bind the eggshell together with an emulsifier (glue), and sell it to the buyer as a natural fortified egg. Will you be buying that egg? Why not buy and consume the real egg rather than a bad imitation of an egg. When you purchase processed food, that is what you are buying, an imitation.

Nutritionist scientists working for food firms are generating unhealthy foods that do not match our biochemistry. They've been able to pinpoint specific molecules that impact our taste buds and brain by experimenting on us with no constraints. They've discovered chemicals that cause our dopamine receptors to crave more of a chemical that leads to food addiction. Flavor enhancers such as sugar and monosodium glutamate (MSG) are two examples of such chemicals. Sugar and MSG are common ingredients in processed foods. When we have a meal of processed foods, no one knows how that soup of different chemicals affects our health and metabolism.

What is ultraprocessed food? For human nutrition, at present, the most salient way to classify foods and drinks is by type, degree, and purpose of processing.[48] When the food industry introduces ingredients and chemicals into a food product that do not naturally occur, it creates a new food matrix that is no longer natural.[10] Ingredients such as refined sugar or high-fructose corn syrup, artificial flavors and colors, preservatives, vegetable oils [2], and emulsifiers are added to make the food's texture more palatable and extend the food's shelf-life. These process techniques fundamentally alter the structure of the food. As a result, we have a completely synthetic product that does not match our human biochemistry.[14]

The NOVA Classification of Food, a brilliant categorization of industrialized human-made food, assigns each food a grade from 1 to 4 based on its degree of processing:

---

[2] From this point forward, we will employ the industry term *vegetable oil* to refer to the refined polyunsaturated oils (fats) from seed and grains used in American kitchens and restaurants for the purpose of cooking.

Group 1. Unprocessed or minimally processed foods

Group 2. Processed culinary ingredients

Group 3. Processed foods

Group 4. Ultraprocessed food and drink products

The categories are explained in more detail in Appendix B.

Some countries are using the NOVA classification for dietary guideline policies. For example, in France, public health nutrition aims to reduce ultraprocessed foods by 20 percent in 5 years. In Brazil, nutritional guidelines recommend limiting the consumption of processed foods and avoiding ultraprocessed foods altogether.[49]

As we have stated and believe is worth reiterating, we have a food technology culture that embraces the assumption that human-made industrialized food can be superior to natural food. Nutrition scientists who work for food companies think that enriching industrialized processed food may provide humans with vital nutrients. What exactly is fortified or enriched food? It is food that has been subjected to a process in which natural nutrients have been removed or substantially removed and substituted with artificial nutrients. The food industry produces refined white flour by grinding and processing raw wheat, removing all nutrients. The original wheat structure has been altered to create a new food matrix that does not match human biochemistry. In the case of margarine, no natural products are used. Margarine is made by the manufacturer using vegetable oil, water, yellow coloring, and occasionally synthetic vitamins. Nutritionism is a term used by Michael Pollan to describe this dietary ideology.[8].The conversion of natural (real) food to processed food has proven unhealthy to humans; it is the cause of today's chronic illnesses.[14]

Processed foods have become commodities and have culminated in ultraprocessed foods. Ultraprocessed foods are unhealthy, sometimes fortified with synthetic vitamins, and usually made of four refined ingredients no longer in a natural state. Those four ingredients are factors contributing to metabolic syndrome:

- Refined grains, usually wheat
- Refined sugars in any of its 252 different designations, including high-fructose corn syrup[13]
- Polyunsaturated fatty acids (PUFAs), high in omega-6 fatty acids, and trans fats that are partially hydrogenated oils
- Cooking with vegetable oils (which used to be considered lubricants for mechanical connections) instead of natural fats

Ultraprocessed foods account for more than 80 percent of the calories consumed in the United States. The percentages are higher in low-income and minority communities. These foods are high in refined sugar and other non-natural chemical ingredients—and they increase the risk of metabolic syndrome.[50]

Ultraprocessed foods are a critical factor that contributes to type 2 diabetes and obesity. People have tried to address the obesity issue with diet and exercise. The ultraprocessed synthetic foods have been engineered to put the appetite into overdrive.[51] You may have noticed the term *artificial flavor* or, sometimes, the more deceiving term *natural flavor*. The two flavors are produced by different methods but contain the same essential chemical compounds.

A chemical industry segment is engaged in the production of synthesizing ingredients for food and beverage flavorings. It develops chemical flavors for all fast-food products, from sugary drinks to ultraprocessed foods sold at fast-food outlets. The processed food industry uses chemical flavors to make its products more palatable and appealing. They also include chemical compounds to give the foods a chewable texture and color. They do this because ultraprocessed foods, whether packaged for sale in grocery stores or sold at fast-food outlets, are unpalatable and must be flavored to taste and look appetizing. This aspect of ultraprocessed food is another reason why we refer to it as industrialized human-made or non-natural. According to Eric Schlosser, today's ultraprocessed foods offer a blank palette. The chemicals you add to them, whatever those chemicals are, give the foods a specific taste and texture.[52]

When confronted with the harmful effect of their food processing and chemicals, food firms unleashed their marketing propaganda and responded with some gimmick that confuses the public. They have recently relied extensively on advertising emphasizing "your right to choose" to appeal to your patriotism. Do you think the food corporations are so egalitarian that they will consider your patriotic interests?[53]

Because their ingredients are cheap and production can be ramped up and down quickly, ultraprocessed foods are the most profitable products of large food companies. Ultraprocessed foods are also one of the leading causes of all metabolic syndrome-related disorders: obesity, type 2 diabetes, high blood pressure, fatty liver, cardiovascular diseases, high cholesterol, cancer, dementia, and other chronic illnesses.[47, 48] According to Michael Pollan, we humans have adapted to many different diets, but the Western diet is not one of them.[8]

For more information on all types of foods and ingredients, one can consult OpenFoodFacts.com, a free online and crowdsourced database listing food products and their ingredients from around the world.

Second Suspect: Sweets and Addictions to Them

Another character is lurking as a suspect: refined sugar. Why refined sugar? Eighty percent of bottled, canned, packaged, or frozen products in supermarkets include added sugar. If you believe you know what sugar is and how to find it in a package, you'll be amazed at how adept the ultraprocessed food business has become in hiding sugar in the ingredients list. According to Dr. Robert

Lustig, the sugar in ultraprocessed meals is hidden behind 252 different designations for sugar.[13, 54]

Take, for example, a situation that made news in 2020. Under Irish law, the bread used in Subway IP, LLC sandwiches do not qualify as bread. Therefore, the government of Ireland is now taxing Subway bread as a pastry. Bread in Ireland should not contain more than 2 percent refined sugar. However, Subway's bread contains 10 percent refined sugar. Subway uses that much sugar in its bread to make its sandwiches more palatable and addictive, as their meats are processed and not particularly healthy or tasty.[55]

At this point in the story, we have to bring back the 1990s Cuban economic crisis. You might not realize it, but Cuba is a major producer of raw sugar cane. Although Cuba's importance as a major export of raw sugar cane has dwindled due to a lack of infrastructure improvements in its sugar mills, the crop remains an essential economic driver. Sugar was so crucial to the Cuban economy that there was a branch of chemistry named "sugar chemistry" (*química azúcarera*) at the University of Havana. Our grandfather studied it at university and worked as a Sugar Master (*Maestro de Azúcar*) in sugar mills in Cuba and Venezuela.

Because our grandfather was a chemist specializing in sugar cane chemistry and processes, we always had a curiosity about sugar cane. Sugar cane is a beautiful perennial grass that grows 6 to 19 feet tall. It is the world's largest crop by production quantity and accounts for 79 percent of refined sugar. The plant has sturdy, jointed, fibrous stalks rich in sucrose which accumulates in the internodes of the stalks. In its raw form, sugar cane can be chewed by peeling the outer layer of the stalk away and masticating the interior wet mass to suck the juice. The liquid juice, called *guarapo*, is made by cold-pressing the sugar cane. Sugar cane juice has a lower glycemic index than refined sugar cane.

Unrefined sugar is a healthy alternative to refined sugar and non-caloric artificial sweeteners (NASs). Randomized research has found that NASs (saccharin, sucralose, aspartame, and acesulfame potassium) may promote obesity-associated metabolic changes by altering the function of the bacteria that colonize the stomach and intestines.[56] Unrefined raw sugar is a whole food; noncentrifugal cane sugar (NCS) is the technical name. This product has not been refined, and therefore, it still contains molasses with all its nutrients. NCS is over 90 percent carbohydrates. Sucrose (sugar) is the predominant carbohydrate (80 percent). NCS also contains calcium, potassium, sodium, chloride, and phosphates and has several other essential nutrients: iron, zinc, magnesium, copper, cobalt, nickel, and chromium.

NCS is known by different names, including unrefined *muscovado, panela, jaggery,* and *rapadura*. NCS should be eaten in moderation; no more than 6 to 9 U.S. teaspoons [3] per day should be consumed. The American Heart Association recommends no

---

[3] A U.S. teaspoon is different than a metric teaspoon. One U.S. teaspoon equals 0.986 metric teaspoon.

more than 9 teaspoons (36 grams) of added sugar per day for men. The figure for women is lower: 6 teaspoons (25 grams) per day and less than 24 grams for children under 18 years.[57] NCS is healthy and nutritious and can sweeten your coffee or tea. Panela, which is our favorite, is a product of Colombia. Many small artisan farmers in that country make a living, crystalizing the *guarapo* (sugar cane juice) into *panela* unrefined organic sugar cane.[58, 59] Do not be deceived by the marketing of products as "organic sugar" or "organic sugar cane" or "organic raw sugar." They are forms of refined sugar marketed to appeal to the consumer. They are not unrefined sugar cane.

You will exceed the recommended number of U.S. teaspoons if you consume packaged or ultraprocessed food containing refined sugar. Consider that a 12-ounce can of soda contains 8 teaspoons (32 grams) of added sugar! In one gulp, you've consumed your entire day's allowance. When sugar is refined in a highly industrialized process, it might be a threat to your health, depending on how much you consume. Over the last 60 years, sugar consumption has skyrocketed to the point that 80 percent of the packaged food items in a grocery store contain sugars. That level of consumption is what makes sugar, whether brown or white, deadly to your health.

Sugar is inherently fattening, according to Dr. Robert Lustig, because it induces insulin resistance. Sucrose is a sugar that includes an equal amount of glucose and fructose. While glucose is disseminated and stored in our cells, fructose is delivered directly to the liver, the only place that it can be metabolized. Fructose, a sugar, is processed in the liver in the same way that alcohol is. Excess fructose is converted to fat in the liver, and too much fructose leads to fatty liver.[6, 46] Insulin resistance is directly affected by liver fat. Insulin resistance leads to elevated insulin levels and type 2 diabetes over time and significantly contributes to obesity.[37]

Fructose is found in fruits, and the fibers in the fruit aid digestion and significantly slow the release of fructose. Fructose in raw fruit does not have the same effect on the liver because the fructose is released slowly into the body and does not overwhelm the liver due to the fruit fiber. In contrast, in fruit juice, the fiber has been removed; thus, fruit juice devoid of fiber is as harmful as a can of sugary beverage.

Third Suspect: Polyunsaturated Vegetable Oils

Refined sugar and ultraprocessed meals have been identified as two suspects, but a third possibility has emerged: seed and grain oils, also known as vegetable oils. Procter & Gamble introduced Crisco shortening, a trans fat made from cottonseeds, in 1911. P&G marketed it as a healthier alternative to the most popular natural cooking fats at the time: lard, tallow, and dairy butter. Crisco oil introduced later, like all vegetable oils, lacks the nutrients found in naturally occurring fats.[5]

Cottonseed oil was the first vegetable oil to be utilized as a lubricant for mechanical connections. However, because manufacturers produced more oil than was required, they promoted it as a "healthy" substitute to natural fats in the kitchen. Have you seen the oil refineries in northern New Jersey, southeastern Texas, or southern California? If you have, you have probably seen a vegetable oil refinery. They are very similar.

During and after the saturated fat controversy in the 1960s and 1970s, the use of vegetable oils skyrocketed. According to Dr. Ancel Keys, who was at the center of the debate, meats and butter contain saturated fat and were blamed for developing cholesterol in the arteries and cardiovascular disorders. As we now know, Ancel Keys' statement about saturated fat could not be proven in his laboratory trials. Therefore, he fed his patients margarine made with partially hydrogenated vegetable oil, a trans fat (not dairy butter). He publicly blamed saturated fat in meats and dairy butter for adverse health effects.[60] Since then, vegetable oils have become a permanent fixture of ultraprocessed cuisines in American kitchens and restaurants, and they are slowly killing us.

Omega-3 and omega-6 fatty acids are found in our cells and are produced from our food. To be healthy, humans require a balance of the two fatty acids. Before introducing seed and grain oils, our forebears omega-6 and omega-3 fatty acids were in a balanced 1:1 ratio. Because of the significant intake of omega-6 found in vegetable oils, the average American omega-6 to omega-3 is a 15:1 ratio, almost seven times the recommended 2:1 ratio.[61] Polyunsaturated fatty acids (PUFAs) are a significant source of fat in our modern American diet because we have eliminated most natural fats. Most vegetable oils (PUFAs) are high in omega-6 fats, which promote inflammation in the body, and are low in omega-3 fats, which reduce inflammation. A balance between the two types is required for our metabolism, and this balance has been lacking in the last 50 years. For example, if you eat salmon, which is high in omega-3 fats, but then fry or boil it in vegetable oil (PUFA), the omega-3 fats will be lost. Individuals that eat that salmon no longer have access to healthy fats.[11]

One of the myths and misconceptions propagated by the food industry and government dietary standards is that PUFAs are good for you, whereas saturated fats are bad. The statement is entirely false. Because their carbons are bonded to hydrogen molecules, saturated fats are more stable than unsaturated fats, which lack some hydrogen bonds. Furthermore, saturated fats, such as dairy butter, are more stable and solid at room temperature because they are more tightly packed. Monounsaturated fats and polyunsaturated fats are the two forms of unsaturated fats. The difference is that mono (one) only has one missing hydrogen link, but poly (many) has many missing hydrogen bonds.

PUFA oils are helpful, according to the industry, because they come from nutritious seeds, grains, and beans, and that is correct; the source is healthy. However, there are two flaws in that assertion. Let's start with a healthy seed like flaxseed, which is full of omega-3 fats in its natural state, and we all know that omega-3 is good for you, right? Yes, flaxseeds are nutrient-dense and high in omega-3 fats at their source. But don't get the flaxseed's origins mixed up with the process of turning it into an oil. Let's have a look at how vegetable oil is made chemically. A solvent is used to extract as much oil as possible from the seed, grain, or bean. One of the commonly used solvents contains hexane, a petrochemical made from crude oil, which is highly hazardous. Once the solvent has extracted the vegetable oil, it is distilled, and heat, steam, and pressure are used to remove the solvent. The oil is not edible at this point; it must be degummed, neutralized, bleached, deodorized, and in some cases, winterized and dewaxed before it can be eaten. The natural flaxseed you started with has been entirely transformed into a wholly artificial product that does not match human biochemistry and no longer includes omega-3 fatty acids.

PUFAs are healthy in their natural state; they are part of cell membranes, which are part of our physiology. PUFAs make up a substantial percentage of the coverings of all our cells. PUFAs also operate as hormone precursors and participate in various signaling pathways, some of which are anti-inflammatory. Therefore, they have numerous advantages. PUFAs, on the other hand, should not be utilized as cooking oil or in other foods because they are not meant to be eaten. They also have a low smoke point [4], making it

---

4 Smoke point occurs when the temperature at which fats in cooking oils begin to degrade and produce smoke as the oil is heated. When oil reaches the temperature at which it begins to smoke, it undergoes a chemical breakdown, resulting in the emission of a gas and other pollutants. Because of this chemical breakdown, the oil may have an unpleasant taste.

easy to heat them to a high temperature beyond the smoke point. When you do that, something in the PUFAs gets damaged, and it becomes pro-inflammatory. So, it's not the food itself that is unhealthy at the source; what we do to process it makes it harmful and lethal.

Vegetable oils have a high omega-6 fat content, which is a problem. Inflammation, heart disease, insulin resistance, and obesity are all linked to high levels of omega-6 fats. Increased use of vegetable oils has been linked to an increase in people dying from heart disease. By 2019, the average amount of vegetable oil used per person per day had climbed to 800 grams, up from 2 grams in 1900.[62] It is easy to see the direct correlation between vegetable oil consumption and heart disease deaths on a graph. In the last 50 years, our consumption of vegetable oils has gone through the roof and so have the number of deaths due to heart disease.[62]

There are more heart disease deaths per year today than in any year from 1900 to 1950. We have reduced saturated fat consumption to the level required by the dietary guidelines, but cardiovascular disease continues unabated. We consume substantially more omega-6 fats in our diet than is healthy for our bodies, while the amount of omega-3 fats has remained constant. The high levels of omega-6 fats that we consume daily have created an imbalance in our biochemistry, causing another condition leading to metabolic syndrome. Like refined sugar, vegetable oils cause fatty liver in approximately 30 weeks of continuous consumption, and vegetable oils are in every processed or fried food product. In obesity studies, vegetable oils are significant contributors to obesity.[63]

A branch of science that studies the effects of fats in the human body is called lipid science. The functions of lipids include storing energy, signaling, and acting as structural components of cell membranes.[64] A brilliant Austrian scientist, Dr. Gerhard Spiteller, has been at the forefront of studying lipids for over 40 years. His seminal work on the subject was published in 2000 and has been cited in many articles about PUFAs and their negative impact on human health.[65]

Dr. Spiteller pointed out that processed vegetable oils (PUFAs) are inherently unstable and are to blame for the hardening of the arteries. The dietary natural saturated fats are not the cause of cholesterol in the arteries. What lipid scientists, such as Dr. Spiteller, have been telling us for years (with support from random research) is that industrially processed vegetable oils are the enemies of your heart and arteries, not natural saturated fats. Vegetable oils impair the absorption of vitamins and do not suppress the appetite.[60]

Vegetable oils are partially hydrogenated fatty acids (trans fats). They have been found to clog the arteries, which is one reason cardiovascular disease continues to rise. One of the early warnings of poor arterial blood flow is erectile dysfunction (ED). ED has been increasing dramatically in the last 50 years, and it may be the proverbial canary in the coal mine, letting us know that arteries are getting clogged. The coronary arteries to the heart may be next.[60]

The industrial-era vegetable oils and spreads that are harmful to your health are the canola, soy, flaxseed, sunflower, cottonseed, grapeseed, corn, safflower oils, and non-dairy butter spreads (including margarine), to name a few. Vegetable oils are ubiquitous in ultraprocessed foods, from fried foods to mayonnaise, salad dressing, and fake olive oil.[60] Many people have touted palm oil as a substitute for vegetable oils. Still, research has found that palm oil is not a safe substitute for partially hydrogenated fats (trans fats) because palm oil results in adverse changes in low-density lipoprotein cholesterol and apolipoprotein B blood concentrations, just as PUFAs (trans fat) does.[66]

The healthy traditional fats are some of the best foods you can eat. They are animal fats (lard, tallow, dairy ghee, and dairy butter) and cold-pressed virgin olive oil.[60] Edible unrefined cold-pressed avocado oil, like extra virgin olive oil, retains the flavor and color characteristics of the fruit flesh. Avocado oil is used for cooking, where it is noted for its high smoke point. A high smoke point is required for frying foods such as French fries. Avocado oil has a fat profile similar to olive oil. When avocado oil is refined for a higher smoke point, it goes through a similar process as PUFAs oils, becoming unhealthy. Unrefined cold-pressed olive and avocado oil are green due to the fruit color. When they are refined and heated, they become yellowish or amber in color. That is how you can tell they are no longer unrefined.

We know from research studies that when polyunsaturated vegetable oils are heated at temperatures required for frying food, oxidation agents are generated that may be dangerous to your health.[5] As the oils oxidize, they become reactive oxygen species, which are highly harmful to our health when exposed to heat, oxygen, light, and pressure (as in a pressure cooker). When we consume them, we cause free radical damage and oxidative stress in our bodies. You are setting loose in your body dangerous particles, and they start damaging your fatty tissues, DNA and proteins, and overall health. Oxidative stress can cause heart disease, hypertension, hardening of the arteries, insulin resistance leading to type 2 diabetes, cancer, and premature aging.[67] When those same oils are heated beyond the recommended heating point, they may give off fumes that contain carcinogens.[60] Most restaurants reuse the same oil for a week or two. They continuously reheat it, creating a hazardous condition for consuming the foods cooked with that reheated oil. A healthy practice is not to order or eat fried food from fast-food outlets or neighborhood restaurants.

Fourth Suspect: Big Brother Is Watching

So, we've identified another suspect in our mystery: vegetable oils. So far, all the suspects identified as being members of the ultraprocessed food gang are processed foods, refined sugar, and vegetable oils. The next suspect is not a food ingredient but a government institution, the U.S. government.

The late U.S. Senator George McGovern chaired the Senate Select Committee on Nutrition and Human Needs, which produced the first dietary goals for the United States in 1977 and the first formal guidelines in 1980. The committee recommended that Americans limit their fat intake to 30 percent of their diet and saturated fat intake to 10 percent.[68] It took until 1992 for the USDA to issue the now-infamous food pyramid. The dietary guidelines promoted carbohydrates as a healthy alternative to meat, dairy products, fish, and other saturated fats. The first pyramid was developed and published in Sweden in 1974 with some controversy. What did the homogeneous Swedish population of 8 million and the heterogeneous American population of 217 million have in common in 1974? The answer is not much, but nonetheless, the U.S. government based its nutritional guidelines on that model. The Swedes stopped using it a few years later.

Dr. Ancel Keys arbitrarily picked 7 countries that suited his theory that saturated fat caused cholesterol buildup and cardiovascular illness based on correlations with only 22 countries investigated.[5, 60] He won the debate in the media and made the cover of *Time* magazine. Cardiovascular diseases were the national obsession back then, and food with saturated fat was blamed for causing them. Because saturated fat resembles cholesterol in the arteries, it was a simple deduction to blame it. Obesity was becoming a concern but was not widespread at that time, so no attention was paid to it. The implications of a high-carbohydrate diet were never publicly addressed. By attempting to solve one health problem, cardiovascular disease, we created an additional health problem, metabolic syndrome, without resolving the original problem.[29]

By establishing dietary guidelines and preventing criticism by some experts, these well-meaning groups of people, along with the food industry, inadvertently reduced good healthy habits and, in a sense, robbed the country of some of its future prosperity. They created a new class of persons in our society, which we now call the metabolic syndrome sick. This group of people is not divided by wealth, poverty, ethnicity, or whether they are blue-collar or white-collar workers. The metabolic syndrome sick goes across all standard social classifications; it includes about half of our population and is expanding.[29]

The ultraprocessed food industry has been trying for years to commoditize food to produce large quantities in centralized factories. The government handed the industry the proverbial keys to the kingdom, so the food companies supported the dietary goals wholeheartedly. The ultraprocessed food companies began to retool and redesign their brightly colored packages, claiming that the foods inside were low fat, reduced fat, nonfat, zero fat, and healthy fat.

In a short period, companies introduced more high-carbohydrate ultraprocessed foods to supermarket shelves than anyone thought possible. They had a problem, however: their processed foods without natural fats tasted like cardboard. They made the foods more palatable by adding refined sugar, artificial flavors, coloring, and texture. Then people could have tasty food and become addicted to it. Biochemists were aware that a high intake of sugar acts like an opioid on our brain's neuroreceptors.[1]

Following the dietary guidelines and consuming the Western diet of ultraprocessed fast food, people got sick and more are getting sick every day. Healthcare expenditures have risen dramatically, diverting public finances from other priorities such as education, infrastructure repair, and defense. Our schools are struggling to deal with our children's obesity, which their peers may mock. At home, the circumstance causes squabbles and blaming among parents. Our citizens are absent from work due to illness, which has hampered national productivity. If half of the population is ill, our national Gross Domestic Products (GDP) suffers.[69]

Obesity increased rapidly after the dietary guidelines were published. Scientists who pointed to research findings contrary to the dogma of the high-carb, low-fat diet were discredited. When research started to show that the saturated fat in natural foods was not the culprit in heart disease, the medical establishment, ultraprocessed food industry, and USDA claimed that research flawed or ignored it.[5]

The reaction to critics of the dietary goals and food pyramid has been an Orwellian overreach. In George Orwell's dystopian novel *Nineteen Eighty-Four*, the Thought Police are employed to discredit individuals and independent thinking.[70] The researchers who questioned the food pyramid dogma were labeled Thought

Criminals in real life because they opposed the establishment's tenets.

The establishment has castigated researchers and doctors that have spoken against the false assumptions of the dietary goals. They are indirectly labeled as Thought Criminals when they point out the detrimental effect on our health of high carbohydrates, including sugar and vegetable oils. If you think we exaggerate, look at what they have done with pizza. It has now been classified as a vegetable and sold in schools because it contains tomato sauce.[71] Isn't that doublethink?

Another aspect of George Orwell's universe in the *Nineteen Eighty-Four* novel is doublethink, which is a method of indoctrination. The government, medical groups, and the ultraprocessed food industry were all guilty of doublethink. A person is encouraged to accept something that is manifestly untrue as true or accept two contradictory beliefs as correct.[70] We can consider the FDA panel members and colleagues who set up the food guidelines as "Big Brother" and doublethink disciples. The FDA and the medical establishment continue to reduce saturated fat in their high-carb, low-fat dietary guidelines. They believe that saturated fat is damaging to cardiovascular health, despite a body of research and data demonstrating that saturated fat does not cause cardiovascular disease.[5] They accept that saturated fat is unhealthy as truth even though it has been proven to be false; this is classic Orwellian doublethink.

The food industry, like the tobacco industry before it, has wrapped itself in health messaging through marketing while continually producing items that are inherently unhealthy, which has had devastating impacts on public health. We assumed that, like in 1984, Big Brother would be the government. However, there is a modern twist. Companies that produce ultraprocessed foods are likewise behaving in a Big Brother-like manner. They use social media and smartphones to follow people's movements, create a marketing strategy, and influence people's decisions regarding food and political matters impacting the sale of ultraprocessed junk food.[72]

You are being bombarded and influenced by advertising on TV, in print, and on social media, and by numerous panels of experts who use doublethink. When a local government seeks to raise taxes on sugary drinks or make the containers for those drinks smaller, the food industry spends a lot of money to convince us that our right to choose is being eroded. Its new marketing slogan is "freedom of choice."[53] It attempts to sway your decision by appealing to your sense of patriotism; therefore, be wary of deceptive advertising practices. The ultraprocessed food industry is at a crossroads, with public and government scrutiny of its activities. As part of its commitment to public health, the industry has the expertise to improve its unhealthy processed foods. Will they? A new chapter in the nation's obesity strategy is about to begin. Will the industry collaborate, or will it unleash an army of lobbyists and become the evil empire?

Fifth Suspect: Food Company Executives

The mystery film is nearing its conclusion, and we have four significant suspects in mind: sugar and its 252 different designations, vegetable oils/trans fats high in omega-6 fats, ultraprocessed fast foods, and the USDA. In this mystery, they are referred to as the "gang of four." Which of the four suspects will turn out to be the bad guy? Are there any additional suspects?

We need to include executives from the top ten food firms in the United States, which control more than 90 percent of the food market. They are aware that they have created a problem, but they are unsure how to solve it. They have empathy for those in bad health, but their business training stops them from seeing the damage they are causing. They are making more unhealthy items to expand their markets and maximize their profits. Whether they realize it or not, they are a part of a functioning society whose industry is only a part.[73] In actuality, they seek to gently distort media communications to persuade people to consume more ultraprocessed fast foods with vegetable oils and sugary drinks. It is a very profitable segment of the market.

Through their ultraprocessed foods and food additives, food companies have contributed to metabolic syndrome and obesity in our society. They must address the underlying causes of their behavior at a level that allows them to change their behavior patterns. A company's culture shapes its behavior, and changing the underlying culture may result in new behavior patterns.[74]

Systemic thinking would encourage company executives to consider their role in the broader society, resulting in long-term solutions rather than short-term problems. Food companies and executives would have to reconsider their mission to provide healthier food for the benefit of both their company and society.

In the short run, food corporations are doing well financially, but they must replace their unhealthy ultraprocessed goods with healthier alternatives. Otherwise, they will follow in the footsteps of the tobacco industry. They had opportunities to avoid going down this road: cigarette firms had only one product; thus, they had no alternatives. We hope they recognize the extraordinary opportunity they now have to help the country and simultaneously help themselves remain a viable and profitable company in the future.

Food and agrochemical firms have an opportunity to rehabilitate themselves by being a positive voice and force in the health debate. It is not a debate about defending their existing food environment. It has been established that their ultraprocessed meals, vegetable oils, refined sugars, and sugary beverages have resulted in a public health calamity.[6, 8, 32, 50, 62, 75] Sustainable agriculture and nutritional food production without unhealthy chemicals and their harmful effects will be vital elements in our near future.[76]

New research is being conducted every day on the detrimental consequences of food corporations' products on the population. Food companies should not be allowed to introduce chemicals into our food supply and profit for the next 50 or 100 years as people die from chronic ailments due to their slow-acting toxic substances. Will corporations rise to the occasion and seek healthy solutions, or will they invest in public relations sloganeers and lobbyists? Ultimately, you might have to face the repercussions of being a villain, as did Purdue Pharma, the maker of OxyContin, which was brought to court on criminal charges and forced to close the company to the detriment of its shareholders.[77] Instead, you may want to seize the opportunity to be a hero and focus on long-term profitability by bringing healthy products to market; small entrepreneurs are already doing so. It is your choice. Choose wisely!

Conclusions

We have come to the end of the film, and now the identity of the villain is no longer a mystery. It just so happens that in this film, there is no one villain but five:

- Ultraprocessed fast foods, sugary beverages, and sugary fruit juices
- Sugar, its 252 different designations, and its companions such as high-fructose corn syrup
- Seed and grain (vegetable) oils with high levels of omega-6 fats that clog our arteries

- The USDA and some medical associations, although redemption is still possible for them if they have the moral fiber to stand against the influence of the food industry
- Food companies and their executives, although redemption is also possible for them if they eliminate the harmful chemicals they add to their products

After this analysis, we conclude that Thomas R. Malthus's theories on population growth and decline due to food abundance and scarcity, respectively, remain relevant today, but they are being realized in unanticipated ways. The Western diet's reliance on ultraprocessed fast foods, vegetable oils, and sugar has exacerbated the incidence of metabolic syndrome diseases, shortening people's lives on the planet. The subsequent population decline will likely be due to an abundance of industrialized unhealthy food, not a lack of food, as Thomas R. Malthus originally predicted.[78]

§ § §

CHAPTER 04.

TWENTY-FIRST CENTURY HEALTH: BOOM OR BUST

> "The world as we have built it is a process of our thinking. It cannot be changed unless we change our way of thinking." Albert Einstein

We need to reassess how the Western diet affects human biochemistry based on the last 50 years of research. Can we eliminate ultraprocessed convenience foods with vegetable oils and sugar, as well as sugary drinks, from our diet? We understand that the current diet is bad for our health, and we need to stop eating it. Are we going to be able to pull it off? It will be difficult. Many medical and food dietitian organizations, government agencies, and food companies are stuck in the late-20th-century paradigm of convenience ultraprocessed foods, unhealthy diets, high carb/low-fat diets, and strict calorie dietary restrictions.

Our population's health has deteriorated for more than 50 years since the dietary guidelines were introduced; meanwhile, type 2 diabetes and obesity are increasing exponentially. Many of you blame it on people who overeat and are not active enough. You do not believe it has much to do with ultraprocessed foods, sugar, or omega-6 fats in vegetable oils, but rather with the amount of food consumed. Let us look at countries where a similar situation has happened in the last 50 years.

While some of you may believe that the world's wealthiest and most developed countries have the highest obesity and type 2 diabetes rates, this is incorrect. Obesity can be found in any country. Some countries, however, have a far higher share than others. The United Nations have identified several countries as having the highest obesity rates. Nauru in the Pacific Ocean has the highest obesity rate, with 61 percent of the population having a body mass index above 30. Nauru's obesity problem, like that of many other South Pacific countries, began when well-meaning Western immigrants taught its people to fry their meals and import less healthy food, abandoning their traditional farming, preparation, and preservation abilities.

After the Pacific island countries, Kuwait has the highest obesity rate in the world, with 38 percent of its people having a body mass index of over 30. The entrance of American fast-food outlets, which have taken over and replaced indigenous food, is faulted for Kuwait's obesity. As a result, diabetes has become more prevalent in Kuwait. It is the same story whenever the Western diet and fast-food outlets are introduced in a country. India and China, both of which are not obese countries, have a greater prevalence of type 2 diabetes today than the United States.[44, 45] The prevalence of type 2 diabetes began to rise in those two countries with the arrival of fast-food outlets and the Western diet. If you still believe that obesity is caused solely by individuals overeating, we have a bridge in Brooklyn that we would like to sell you; in other words, your conclusion is wrong.

Despite these facts, the food industry in the United States has a strong lobby in Washington, D.C. that works to undermine any efforts to link food companies to our health crisis. Furthermore, food corporations continue to introduce more unhealthy products to enhance their sales and profits. The general public, particularly low-income employees and minorities, are the primary consumers of ultraprocessed foods. The snack food business is so lucrative that some companies solely make snacks and convenience meals composed of synthetic components with no natural ingredients. Yet, they have the audacity to sell their unhealthy products as "healthy snacks." They are available on many school grounds and in hospitals recommended by the dietitians in those institutions.

Sugar, as previously stated, is the worst product because it contains 50% fructose, which is metabolized in the liver. Cirrhosis or fatty liver can be caused by alcohol, which is also metabolized in the liver. Counting the calories in sugar without first understanding the biochemistry of how fructose affects our organs is irresponsible.[6] In response to the carbohydrates and sugar consumed, the pancreas secretes insulin. Too much sugar can lead to a fatty liver, which causes the pancreas to produce more insulin, resulting in insulin resistance. Insulin resistance is a hormonal imbalance that leads to type 2 diabetes. Dr. Jason Fung asserts that type 2 diabetes is not like every other known disease. Type 2 diabetes has a unique and malignant potential to devastate our entire body. Practically no organ system remains unaffected by diabetes.[24]

Can we prevent or reverse insulin resistance and type 2 diabetes? The good news is that yes, we can. How? You need to understand that the disease is food-related. The disease starts when we adopt a high-carbohydrate, ultraprocessed convenience food diet prepared with vegetable oils and added sugar. We can prevent it and reverse it when choosing a healthier green vegetable diet with healthy natural meats and fats. Metabolic syndrome and its disorders are, for the most part, food-related illnesses, and they can usually be reversed by eating healthy food and making lifestyle changes.[29] The Cuban experience is proof of that statement. If you are prediabetic or have type 2 diabetes, diabetes can be reversed, but the damage it has already caused to your organs, such as the kidneys, cannot be reversed. However, the longer you wait to cure your diabetes, the more harm to your organs.

How Food Companies Are Hacking Your Mind

Robert Lustig, MD, has written a superb book, *The Hacking of the American Mind*.[72] He explains how food companies have manipulated our desires using biochemistry to market harmful products with the FDA's tacit approval. Lustig asserts that there has been an epidemic of negative extremes over the last four decades: addiction (from excessive pleasure) and despair (from not enough happiness). During that time, our understanding of neuroscience has evolved to the point that these two emotions can now be deconstructed and analyzed at a biochemical level. He describes how our pursuit of happiness leads to a food-addiction culture, which eventually leads to despair. He explains how our needs and desires for happiness affect our brains in chemical terms.

Dopamine is a neurotransmitter that tells the brain that ingesting a substance makes you feel good and that consuming more will make you feel even better until you get hooked. Marijuana and cocaine are two examples of such substances. Sugar promotes the release of dopamine, and the more sugar we consume, the more we crave it, whether it's in the form of sugary drinks, fruit juices, cookies, sweets, or ultraprocessed foods. Serotonin is a neurotransmitter that tells our brains that we are happy and satisfied and do not require an additional substance. According to Dr. Lustig, dopamine produces a short-term joyful feeling that leaves you wanting more; serotonin, on the other hand, delivers longer-lasting feelings of satisfaction or contentment that prevent the desire for more of a substance.

Corporations have used "neuromarketing" to persuade customers to purchase their goods and experience the desired pleasure. This type of marketing evaluates people's brain responses to company advertisements, eliminating the guesswork associated with previous marketing techniques.[72] When a product induces the release of dopamine, the user becomes tolerant of the substance and requires more, which is the effect of a narcotic drug. The food industry is so confident about the dopamine response that it advertises ultraprocessed snacks as irresistible, daring you to consume just one—obese individuals often complain about how difficult it is to change their eating habits.

Science Versus Dogma?

As we noticed when researching the public health issue, one of the observations was a schism (split) in the scientific community. A new generation of doctors and scientists has formed their beliefs on empirical, pragmatic evidence. They are implementing effective measures that work and are not confined by outdated dogmas and half-truths that have resulted in an ill and dying population.[9] Most government organizations and established institutions are preoccupied with old hypotheses and soft ideologies with little or no basis in physical reality or science.

The health crisis has compelled this new breed of doctors, scientists, and educated people to reconsider their fundamental beliefs. They are discovering that many of those earlier precepts were not entirely correct and too limited in scope. Now that these professionals are broadening their perspectives, the future appears brighter and more receptive to viable ideas.

It is true that ultraprocessed, unhealthy food makes us sick and even kills us prematurely. So, why hasn't the government declared ultraprocessed foods to be dangerous to your health? We are much closer to the Malthusian world than we would like to accept, not because of the traditional population cycle of increase and decline that Malthus predicted but because of the unexpected reduction in life expectancy due to the abundance of unhealthy ultraprocessed food.[79, 80]

Government for the People?

We must wonder why our government is so slow to react to health issues affecting the general public. We understand that in our democracy, corporations have the right to be heard. However, when that right is abused by those who make political campaign contributions and lobbyists who use delaying tactics while the population suffers, it is time to do something about it. But first, let us look at the slow actions of our government: Following, we offer a condensed version of various government reactions to major public health issues. Appendix C discusses these issues in more detail.

Asbestos. Foreign countries have either banned asbestos outright or issued legislation to protect their people from it for almost 90 years. The United States has not banned asbestos, and its standards that have been legislated are ineffectively enforced.

Lead paint. Foreign countries banned lead in paints early in the 20th century. In an unprecedented move by a corporation, Sherwin-Williams reported the dangers of paint containing lead in a July 1904 company publication, noting that a French expert had deemed lead paint dangerous to the public. Even after that admission by a major paint manufacturer, it took the U.S. government 74 years to ban the substance.

Lead Gasoline. In 1924, the Ethyl Gasoline Corporation began to produce and market TEL (a lead additive to gasoline). In the first 2 months of its operation, the new plant was plagued by cases of lead poisoning, hallucinations, and insanity, and five workers died. The New Jersey state authorities stopped production of the product until safety standards were put in place. In 1973 the EPA mandated a phased-in reduction of lead content in all grades of gasoline. In 1974 the EPA required at least one grade of unleaded gasoline for new 1975 vehicles. Finally, in 1996 the EPA banned leaded fuel for on-road vehicles (sales of leaded gasoline were only 0.6 percent of all gasoline sales by that year.) It was an empty gesture by the EPA. The U.S. government knew in 1924 that lead was poisonous and hazardous to humans. Still, it took 72 years to ban it as an additive to gasoline for road vehicles and then only issue a ban when the sales were practically nonexistent.

Cigarette smoking and vaping. It took the U.S. government 12 years to issue a weak warning on packs of cigarettes and another 25 years to issue a stronger warning after states sued the tobacco companies.

A current version of smoking is vaping. In 2019 and 2020, an outbreak of severe lung diseases due to vaping in the United States was strongly linked by the Centers for Disease Control and

Prevention (CDC) to the vitamin E acetate in vaping products. The government is reviewing the case, and it has not reached a committee in Congress yet.[81]

Trans fats. As early as 1956, studies in the scientific literature showed that trans fats could cause a significant increase in coronary artery disease. After 5 decades, however, the concerns were still primarily unaddressed. Finally, in 2015, the FDA determined that partially hydrogenated oils (PHOs) are not Generally Recognized as Safe (GRAS) and removed them from the GRAS list of substances that are considered safe to add to food (see Appendix C for more information). To allow the food industry time for reformulation, the agency changed the original date of compliance. It gave the industry until 2021 for products containing PHOs to work their way through the distribution system.[82] It was a tacit admission by the FDA that a PHO is a toxin. The FDA finally acted after more than 50 years after lipid researchers had sounded the alarm.

These are just some significant situations where the U.S. government was slow to act in the public interest. Is this going to be the case with the ultraprocessed food industry? For over 50 years, our consumption of ultraprocessed food has increased. Unfortunately, so has the incidence of metabolic syndrome diseases such as type 2 diabetes, obesity, cardiovascular disease, cancer, and dementia, to name a few. How much longer do we have to wait to get, at a minimum, a warning label on the packages of processed food and containers of sugary beverages?

The following chapters may provide a solution that will benefit people and take the place of our slow-acting government in making effective changes in the current unhealthy food environment.

§ § §

Chapter 05.

Unhealthy Food and the Free Market Economy

Americans have begun to eat healthier in the last few years, but the percentage that eats healthier is still small and consists of small demographics. Some companies have joined that trend by providing more wholesome and nutritious foods, such as Whole Foods, Fresh Markets, and real food restaurants, and we commend their efforts. They still sell some food products that contain harmful compounds, however.

Unhealthy ultraprocessed foods and fast-food outlets are not going away. In our democracy, we will have difficulty regulating them, but something needs to be done, especially with growing food delivery services to the home. The food environment impacts our most vulnerable citizens, the low-income service workers, and minorities who patronize fast-food outlets because they are affordable.

We eat more ultraprocessed foods, vegetable oils, and refined sugar than at any other period in history, as described in Chapter 3. It may not be harmful to our health to eat those products occasionally or on a festive occasion. The problem is that we overconsume them since they are cheap, abundant, addictive, and convenient to eat. Sometimes we have no option, such as consuming vegetable oils because they have entirely replaced all-natural cooking fats. The recommended daily allowance for refined sugar, for example, is 6 U.S. teaspoons a day.[57] We consumed an average of 25 U.S. teaspoons every day or around four times more than is recommended. You might say we are doing this because it's our choice, but you would also have to ask whether we have enough information to know how much sugar we are eating. In supermarkets, 80 percent of the packaged foods contain sugar, which is not identified on many nutritional labels. We have no means of finding out how much sugar we consume daily, and this gives us no control over our intake.

The food industry adds sugar to processed foods to make them more palatable and addictive. Sugar's addictive nature causes people to buy and eat more, unaware of how much sugar they consume because of the difficulty of counting how much sugar is in processed food. The same can be said for vegetable oils. We stopped consuming natural fats and substituted them with vegetable-oil-derived fats. Everything we prepare and cook nowadays uses vegetable oils, whether in our kitchens, fast food outlets, or restaurants. Vegetable oil is so ubiquitous that it is practically impossible to eat a meal without the oil. The food industry claims that we have a choice, but we don't when the food industry and the government are complicit in concealing what they do to the processed food we eat.

On grocery store shelves and in restaurants, processed foods with unhealthy ingredients outnumber natural food options. The FDA does not regulate processed food products under existing FDA criteria if they are not immediately toxic. Even if a product has the potential to be hazardous in the long run, the FDA will not regulate it or delay a resolution for decades. We can cite trans fats, which were finally banned after more than 50 years of research demonstrating that they clogged the arteries. The FDA had no choice; the evidence was unmistakable. The FDA never considered labeling the package with a warning. As a result, we must use an example unrelated to the food industry to demonstrate why ultraprocessed foods should be regulated.

Tobacco products are a prime example. The effect of smoking one cigarette per week was not highly damaging, but because smoking is addicting, individuals smoked one or two packs, or 10 to 20 cigarettes, every day. This level of consumption proved to be toxic and lethal. Despite all the evidence indicating how deadly cigarette smoking is for humans, the U.S. Congress had trouble regulating it. All they could do was put a warning label on the package. The states successfully initiated legal action against tobacco firms to collect the health costs of cigarette smoking. They also raised the sales tax on cigarettes. Unfortunately, sales taxes differed between states' jurisdictions, introducing a new challenge of interstate cigarette smuggling.[83]

We now have the same toxicity problem with ultraprocessed foods, vegetable oils, and refined sugar as we formerly had with cigarettes. Therefore, it is about time for ingredient labels to be upgraded with more meaningful advice identifying what has been done to the processed food. A label classification like NOVA will be beneficial. The nutrition label should also include the recommended daily allowance for granulated sugar of 6 to 9 U.S. teaspoons (24 to 36 grams). Total sugars should be identified on the label, including the 252 sugar designations. Also, a cautionary label should be placed prominently on the packaging of all ultraprocessed foods, similar to the one used on cigarette packages.

Free Market Uncontrolled Business Behavior

What are the root causes of this unhealthy food environment? In Chapter 3, we have described the suspects and environment in which this health calamity has been allowed to emerge. To understand the root causes, we need to investigate business behavior and our free-market economy. To illustrate business behavior, let's look at an example at the turn of the 20th century.

While working in a sanitarium in Michigan, Dr. Kellogg hit upon his famous corn flakes. He and his brother formed a company to produce and sell the product. The product became very popular, and in a few years, there were entrepreneurs and other food companies competing with similar products. Competitors needed to differentiate their products, and they began to make the cereals sweeter by adding more sugar. Of course, Kellogg's company had to respond and create frosted corn flakes, adding more sugar. As a business in a growing market, the food companies began to develop more sweet breakfast products. They wanted to expand the market and advertised heavily to children appealing to their sweet palate and making them addicted to sugar at an early age. We have known for over 70 years that consuming sugar is not healthy for humans, and it is addictive.

When businesses discover growing markets, competitors jump into the fray. Usually, a new business can get ahead of an established competitor by differentiating its product in the market. In the food industry, it is difficult to add value to a food product. Food companies compete in price, make the product more palatable (adding unhealthy sugar and chemicals), or make meaningless marketing claims that appeal to customers. Once a competitor finds a way to increase its market share, there is a feeding frenzy; the other food companies use a similar strategy to compete. It fosters aberrant conduct in corporations and their management, hurting their consumers and lying to authorities to protect their harmful products. Unfortunately, we have seen this type of conduct in the executives of large corporations much too often. To mention a few, the tobacco industry, asbestos industry, gasoline additive manufacturers, automobile companies, and recently pharmaceutical companies are all guilty of this behavior. The public and regulators are fed up with those industry's tactics, and they are starting to bring criminal charges and imprison company executives.

A businessperson's concerns are whether the market is growing, their product sales are increasing, competitors are introducing new products, and the products are profitable. Business people know that they will not last as corporate executives or have a viable business if they do not grow sales and make greater and greater profits every year. Therefore, they need to keep introducing more profitable food products into the market to attract more customers. The most profitable food products are the ultraprocessed, convenience sugary products. They are industrially produced products that can be manufactured and distributed relatively quickly and in large quantities. Because the products are not considered toxic (poison), the government has no reason to regulate them under its guidelines. Hence our health calamity has been created by the abundance of chronically toxic, harmful, and addictive ingredients added to our food supply. Our government is aware of the toxicity but does not regulate it due to pressure from the food companies.

Suppose the government does not have the will to use the regulatory avenue, whether federal or state, but the government can tax unhealthy products. It can apply those taxes towards remedying our health calamity of chronic metabolic syndrome diseases. The tobacco industry is again an excellent example of suing for recovery of health costs through taxation. To deal with the health calamity, we will present in Chapter 12 a new form of product taxation for unhealthy foods and the economic concept of disvaluing.

We need to feed a growing global population. The U.S. population will grow by 100 million people in the next 50 years, so it will be necessary to feed a nation of 430 million. We need expertise and investments in agricultural products and processed nutritious food without added chemicals, empty sugar calories, or synthetic vegetable oils. Food companies know how to create nutritional products without adding artificial compounds. Small entrepreneurs are already coming out with those products. Why wait? Food companies need to employ systemic thinking tools to achieve new objectives and generate new company cultures.[74, 84] Their survival and future as viable food companies depend on those actions. Remember, Perdue Pharma.

§ § §

CHAPTER 06.

NATURAL (REAL) FOOD: AN AMERICAN PARADOX

In our real-life story, we have identified the villains: the Western diet of ultraprocessed foods and their additives, food industry practices in manufacturing the foods, and government policies that allow it. Next, we'll discuss natural (real) food, eating behavior, and the benefits of eating healthy. We are not talking about the many diets focused on calories that claim to help you lose weight. Those diets, while initially beneficial, do not work in the long run. That is the American paradox: we have exercised and attempted to eat healthily, but we remain overweight.

The paradox is found in the convenience foods we buy at supermarkets and restaurants. Although we think they are healthy and nutritious, they are really harmful ultraprocessed foods. Most consumers do not read beyond the bold letters on the package and are deceived by the marketing claims (see Chapter 3). There are numerous healthy claims on the box or wrapper in bold, bright lettering. Some examples include low-calorie, low-fat, no-calorie, natural fruit juice, high-fiber vegan, dairy-free, low-sugar, and healthy snacks. Natural flavors (the result of numerous harmful chemicals) and other additives are found in practically all products. We know that processed foods cause diabetes, obesity, and other illnesses, but what can we do about it? We are going to explore that question.

Should We Go Back to Being Prehistoric Humans?

According to anthropologists and archeologists, the earliest *Homo sapiens* (modern humans) were foragers in hunter-gatherer groups or tribes.[85, 86] These tribes lived on plants, roots, and berries found on the land; today, we call them *organic vegetables* or *fruits*. They also hunted for meat when animals migrated into their territory. Today, we call those meats *pasture-raised meats*. Homo sapiens consumed the whole animal, including the organs. Some nomad tribes migrated with the animals, and their food was mostly meat.

We mention this because we assume that modern humans cannot reproduce the hunter-gatherer diet today. The best way to interpret that early diet for our times is that pasture-raised meat and organically raised green vegetables and fruits promote health and longevity. However, we don't know all the aspects of the original diet.[16] Plants and animal meats have been part of the human diet since prehistoric times. The nutrition and survival of early humans depended on the land and good weather for plants to grow.[85]

Prehistoric humans spent a vast amount of time searching for food because they did not have the means to store it. There were periods of abundance and scarcity.[86] Until the agricultural revolution, scarcity of food was part of the human condition. Here we will discuss the time of abundance; the time of scarcity is discussed in Chapter 7.

Foods That Promote Health and Reverse Disease

In the 1950s and 1960s, an alarming number of Americans were dying of heart disease. They were primarily adult men in the later years of life. U.S. Senator George McGovern headed a committee that developed and published the dietary goals in 1977 and dietary guidelines in 1980, later becoming the infamous food pyramid. The guidelines introduced a low-fat, high-carbohydrate diet but did not consider the diet's implications for the population, and consequently, they created a new health problem.[5, 9]

We have an abundance of food choices in this country. We need to make the right food choices because they have significant consequences for our health. It would help if you were not confused when entering a supermarket with tens of thousands of food products. Natural (real) food is available, but it may not be seen in the center aisles. Real food may not have the glittering packaging of ultraprocessed foods with health claims prominently displayed on them. Real food is in all the rainbow's colors and is usually found in the far corners or back aisles of the supermarket. We should not forget the minimally processed foods, including dry legumes such as black, white, red, and pink beans, garbanzo beans, and lentils.[87] Those foods have not lost their nutrients with the drying process.

A healthy diet is straightforward to follow if you eat real food, that is, foods you buy at a farmers' market or in the supermarket's produce or meat section. Meat is full of nutrients and healthy fats. The saturated fat in meats and dairy products is healthy and does not cause a spike in blood sugar, as does food high in carbs.[5, 88] The colors of vegetables, pulses (legumes or beans), tubers, and fruits usually indicate their nutrients.[8] As we said, they are like the colors of the rainbow, enticing and natural.

Organic green leafy vegetables, fruits, pasture-raised meats, and wild fish will give you the nutrients you need for a healthy lifestyle. Your metabolism has had millions of years to adapt to digesting these nutrients. Eat what is natural and drink water. You may consume raw fruits in moderation. The fructose in fruits is another form of sugar, and the fruits need to be consumed in their raw, unaltered form to avoid spikes in blood sugar. Raw fruits contain fiber that is digested and slows the process to get to your bloodstream. Do not consume fruits as juices or smoothies; fruit juices and making a smoothie concentrate the fructose (sugar), which causes spikes in blood sugar, and consequently can be dangerous if you are prediabetic or have type 2 diabetes.

In his new book *Metabolical*, Dr. Robert Lustig mentioned that the food you eat should protect your liver and feed your gut. Natural (real) food does that; ultraprocessed foods do not. Ultraprocessed foods become toxic after being processed and stripped of their natural nutrients and having chemicals added that are harmful to human health.[13] There are many excellent books and cookbooks on the benefits of a natural diet include organic vegetables, fruits, pasture-raised meats, pasture-raised dairy foods, and wild-caught fish—in other words, real food. Do not be influenced by the advertising claims for "natural superfoods." There are no superfoods; it is a marketing gimmick. Natural foods are entirely healthy. No single food type will give you all the nutrients required by your body. You obtain the nutrients necessary for health by eating a variety of natural foods.

One key factor in the Cuban health results was the evidence that eating a diet of green vegetables, healthy meats, and fats (occasionally), and wild-caught fish (when available) was beneficial. Also, avoiding sugary beverages and ultraprocessed foods with sugar and vegetable oils was essential to decrease chronic metabolic syndrome diseases. Of course, we cannot ignore the fact that the Cubans ate only one or two meals a day, did not eat any snacks, did not eat any food on some days, and were very physically active. We understand these results came from a country in crisis, but we can generally conclude that those factors were beneficial to most Cubans in achieving their extraordinary results.

Let us be clear: there is no such thing as a one-size-fits-all diet. At the very least, a diet should be personalized to a person's underlying health conditions, age, and gender. Nevertheless, we can state with certainty that the Western diet does not match our biochemistry and is therefore unsuitable for humans.[6, 8, 51] "Do not eat what a human hand has made; eat what the hand of God provides," a preacher who was an enthusiastic natural food supporter declared in a church sermon. That is sound advice for consuming natural (real) foods in general.

Although almost all nutritional experts with biochemistry training agree that you should eat natural food, they do not agree on the type of food. This is understandably so because we are all physiologically different. One certainty is that all-natural foods are healthy and good to eat. Some people may be allergic to a specific food compound, whereas other people are not. Some people gain weight from certain foods but others do not.

Recent research on the personalized effects of a particular food on an individual implies that foods affect us differently. The data indicate that we, as individuals, are the variable to consider. A specific food can be detrimental to one individual, be beneficial to another, or affect a third person differently.[89-91] This hypothesis represents a new paradigm for nutritional and health benefits. We can minimize or maximize the metabolic effects of foods on an individual by knowing which foods are beneficial for that individual. The individual becomes the variable to study.[90] Eventually, checking an individual's nutritional needs and how they affect their metabolism should be like going to the doctor for your annual visit. It will be part of the blood panel test.

You may have asked yourself, what should I eat? You may not need to follow a specific diet if you are a healthy individual. If you are healthy, you may experiment with different natural (real) foods. But if you are allergic to some foods or believe that you may be allergic to a particular food, avoid it and consult a nutritionist who understands biochemistry. If you have any underlying condition such as type 2 diabetes, obesity, or other illnesses, you may need a personalized diet. Remember that whenever you choose food that is right for you, make sure it is natural (real) food and not human-made (ultraprocessed convenience) food.

Many diet books describe how different diets have helped people avoid disease and lose weight.[9, 17, 92-94] There is no single diet appropriate for everyone; we are individuals with physiological differences. These differences are the primary reason that a healthy diet should be personalized. When it comes to a personalized diet, the variable is the person, not the food.

§ § §

CHAPTER 07.

A TIME TO EAT AND A TIME NOT TO EAT

So far, we have discussed **what not to eat** and **what to eat**. Next, we will discuss the **time to eat** and the **time not to eat** at all.

According to Dr. Jason Fung, long-term weight loss is a two-step process.[95] Usually, our focus is to eat less of certain foods to lose weight. We also need to consider insulin resistance, however. Why insulin resistance? As we previously discussed, insulin resistance is caused by consuming unhealthy ultraprocessed foods containing vegetable oils and refined sugar.

The processed food companies are so good at manipulating our desires through marketing and manufacturing palatable foods that we cannot distinguish healthy from unhealthy food. In addition to processed convenience foods, they have created an ultraprocessed food category called "healthy snacks" (think unhealthy snacks) prepared with vegetable oils and added sugar. Because we snack throughout the day, we eat 7 to 10 times per day rather than 3 times per day. There is no longer a "mealtime." We have become an eating machine all day long. Our metabolism does not rest, and we produce more insulin to compensate for the increase in sugary food. This continuous stimulation of insulin leads to insulin resistance, type 2 diabetes, and obesity.

Choosing Times to Eat?

What is time-restricted feeding? It is a specific method for scheduling mealtimes. We need to break the behavior of constantly eating. One proven benefit is to restrict how many times you eat during the day. You can eat three times, two times, or one time a day; a structured schedule helps your metabolism. For example, if you have dinner at 7:00 pm, you don't have to have anything to eat until breakfast at 7:00 am the next day. You have restricted the time you do not eat by 12 hours; then, you have three meals in the next 12 hours. If you were to continue this effort by skipping breakfast the next day and did not eat until lunchtime at 11:00 am, that would be a 16-hour restricted eating cycle. Afterward, you could eat twice in the next 8 hours. There is also a 24-hour cycle, or one meal a day (OMAD). You have dinner at 7:00 pm and don't have anything to eat, other than water, coffee, or tea (no milk or sugar), until the next day at 7:00 pm, which is dinnertime. The time-restricted feeding cycle reestablishes the circadian rhythms of our bodies. This method has been used successfully to reduce weight and prevent and reverse type 2 diabetes.

What is fasting? We can call fasting the antithesis of a diet. To be on a diet, you must eat food, but you do not eat while fasting.

Humans have been fasting for millennia. In prehistoric times they fasted because of a lack of food storage options, and later they fasted for spiritual reasons as they became urbanized. Eastern and Western religions have certain days of the year or month on which they practice fasting.[96] The era of classical Greece lasted for approximately 200 years during the fifth and fourth centuries B.C.E. In Greek culture, fasting became a social norm. From Socrates to Plato, the Greeks believed that fasting sharpened the mind, which was good for a healthy body. There are records of Greek scholars requesting that their students fast before attending classes. Their rationale was that students were more alert and their minds sharper after fasting. Hippocrates of Cos, a Greek physician who lived in the classical period, recommended that corpulent (overweight) people eat only one meal a day and fast the rest of the day. We may consider fasting as the first diet in recorded history.

Fasting has been part of the evolution of *Homo sapiens*. Early humans did not have food regularly, and they had no means of storing food for times of scarcity.[86] Prehistoric people spent an excessive amount of time foraging food to eat, and depending on the season and the weather, food was not always available.[85, 86] Nature provided a way for the human body to store energy in the form of fat, however. For early humans, this was a blessing. That energy reserve (fat) allowed them to hunt or gather food after not eating for days.

With the abundance of food today, that biological fat storage has become a curse. We eat too much and the wrong kind of food.

During the Industrial Revolution in the early 19th century, workers ate twice a day. Sometime in the first half of the 20th century, we began to eat breakfast, lunch, and dinner. As our society became more mobile with automobile travel and paved roads in the 1950s, cheap food became available in fast-food outlets along highway intersections, and our eating behavior began to change. At first, fast food was reasonably healthy, but it began to change as food companies began centralizing food production at factories for efficiency.[97] Food was prepared for a long shelf-life with added chemical preservatives and partially hydrogenated (trans fat) vegetable oils and was shipped to fast food restaurants for sale to consumers.[98] Fast food became ultraprocessed and unhealthy. Around the late 1970s and early 1980s, there was an explosion of the processed foods we call ultraprocessed fast foods today. The food was marketed as healthy and convenient. The metabolic syndrome and obesity generation was beginning to emerge.

We have already discussed a healthy diet and its benefits for curing and reversing chronic diseases, including cardiovascular disease. What about fasting? What are its benefits? Can we stop eating? Primitive religions and more sophisticated cultures such as the Greeks and the Romans knew about the benefits of fasting, and they practiced it regularly.[18] In 1911 Upton Sinclair published a book on fasting, including the benefits of fasting. Sinclair practiced fasting regularly. He experienced hunger the first day, barely hungry by the second day, and not hungry by the third day. Sinclair recommended that people fast for about 12 days or until hunger returns.[99] You may want to start slow and work your way up to longer fasts. Extreme and extended fasts like 12 days are not required to reverse diabetes or obesity. It is a personal choice. Consult a physician before embarking on any diet, especially if you take any medication or have underlying health issues.

Usually, people ask, why not just lower your food intake? The problem with low caloric intake is that it makes you always feel hungry. Sinclair explained that phenomenon in his book. We discovered later in the century that the reason for hunger is that your metabolism adapts to the lower intake of calories. Therefore, you do not get the benefits of fasting. One of the advantages of fasting is the healthy entry into the state of ketosis, a physiological condition in which your metabolism switches from burning carbohydrates to burning fat for energy. Diets that produce ketoses are popular methods for losing weight.

Modern research shows that fasting has the following benefits: it enhances mental clarity and concentration, induces weight and body fat loss, improves the burning of metabolic fat, lowers blood sugar levels, reduces blood pressure, improves insulin sensitivity (lowering insulin resistance), reduces cholesterol levels, decreases inflammation, and improves metabolic function.[100] Fasting is the most natural "diet" because it is simple: do not eat. Our prehistoric body is "programmed" for fasting. With fasting, you not only lose weight plus gain all the benefits mentioned above, but you also save a lot of money. Give it a try. What do you have to lose but a few pounds and a few diseases? However, we stress in the strongest terms that it is wise to consult with your physician before starting any diet or fasting program.

Personal Experience with Fasting

We are in an excellent place to share my (Emilio, Jr.) experience with intermittent fasting. At the beginning of the book, I told you that I would update you on my chronic diseases. Well, here it is. I spent a few weeks in the south a few summers ago visiting my father. I discovered that he had been fasting for 24 hours three times a week for 3 months and had lost 14 pounds. He also walked 2 miles every day. All of his vital signs had improved. While I was visiting him, he suggested that I try intermittent fasting as a diet. He recommended that I read Dr. Jason Fung's book *The Obesity Code*, and after reading it, I decided to attempt fasting.[24]

My monthly routine began with a week of time-restricted eating (I went without food for 16 hours with an 8-hour feeding period), one meal a day (OMAD) for a week (24-hour fasting), and a fasting period of 48 hours (once a week for 2 weeks.) I checked my blood sugar, which had dropped somewhat, and my blood pressure, which had fallen significantly during the day. I continued to take my prediabetes, high blood pressure, cholesterol, and other medications.

Fasting was simple. However, I did get a little hungry on fasting days during the first week. By the second week, I was no longer hungry. So, 3 weeks after starting my 24-hour fast, I decided to do a 48-hour fast the next day. I was a little hungry at the end of the 24 hours, but I felt like I could handle the next 24 hours, so I took my meds and went to bed. Then, at about midnight, I awoke feeling sick to my stomach; my head was spinning, I had no energy, fainted a couple of times, and couldn't get out of bed. We dialed 911, and my blood pressure was 90/50 mm Hg when the paramedics arrived and took my vitals. I was transported to the nearest hospital, which was only a couple of miles away. The doctors discovered that fasting had dropped my blood pressure and that lisinopril (medication that lowers high blood pressure) had reduced it further. After an overnight stay, I was released from the hospital. My lisinopril dosage was cut from 30 mg to 2.5 mg. I shared this story to warn you to be cautious and consult your doctor before beginning a fasting program, as I should have done. Furthermore, I want you to know that although fasting has many benefits, it might be dangerous if you take any drugs.

After I returned to my home in the north, I contacted my physician, who was amazed by the initial promising results of my fast: I had lost 12 pounds in 4 weeks. I continued fasting, but this time under the supervision of my physician. I've lost 42 pounds after 10 months of fasting and eating real food; my A1C (blood sugar) is now in the normal range; my blood pressure is now stable at 115/70 mm Hg, and my cholesterol has been dropping slowly, however. I'm no longer pre-diabetic or have high blood pressure, and I'm not taking any metabolic syndrome medications. I'm not only saving money on meds but also on meals. It is the easiest and cheapest diet I have ever followed, based on my own experience. I can attest that fasting has helped me lose weight and eliminate several metabolic syndrome conditions. Fasting activates specific hormonal changes, according to research.[37, 101] These hormonal changes do not happen with caloric reduction.

Fasting lowers insulin levels, which helps to prevent insulin resistance and maintains a high metabolic rate. Glucose and fat are the body's energy sources, as we know. There is a myth that fasting causes muscle loss. However, this is not true. Excess glucose is stored as fat in our cells, and the absence of food leads the stored fat to be used as fuel to keep us going, resulting in weight loss. In addition, fasting causes the body's insulin production to decrease.

§ § §

CHAPTER 08.

COVID-19: LESSONS FROM UNHEALTHY COMMUNITIES

When we started to see and hear the first news coming from China in January 2020 about the coronavirus, it appeared that the virus was only present in China. Then it began to emerge in Europe and the United States. We hunkered down at home and watched the news with apprehension. Like everyone else, we saw the pandemic unfolding and the human statistics being gathered on the virus.

Initially, the CDC was concerned mainly about the high mortality rate among the elderly. Also, people with chronic diseases appeared to be more vulnerable to the virus. It was disconcerting for me (Emilio, Jr.) because of my underlying conditions at the time. Although I'm not that old, it was stressful. People with type 2 diabetes were more likely to have severe complications. One reason is that high blood sugar weakens the immune system, and people with a compromised immune system are less able to fight off bacterial and viral infections.[37]

When more details of the mortality statistics became known, it was evident that minorities were being affected the most, especially African Americans, Latinos or Hispanic Americans, and Native

Americans.[25] Early explanations by politicians and the press did not make sense. The reality is that those communities are made up of low-income or poor people, with large (usually multigenerational) families living in very crowded conditions and having little if any healthcare. They also tend to eat an inexpensive diet of ultraprocessed foods.

Service workers are critical to the smooth running of our economy and society at large, and they are on the front line services for the public. Because they faced the public and were willing to do their jobs during the pandemic, they also were at the highest risk of contracting the virus.[102] For the first time, a pandemic made us recognize how crucial they are to our society and economy, and we now refer to them as "essential workers." We needed a pandemic to make us realize how important they are to our economy. We were upset by the way the virus was affecting these hard-working Americans. Their plight was another inspiration for including solutions to their situation in this book.

In some ways, the Covid-19 epidemic is like the national Cuban health crisis. We could all learn from it that healthier people would have fared better against the virus, especially our minorities and low-income people. Covid-19 was our nation's epiphany. The disease hit minorities and the poor dramatically because of their underlying health issues, which resulted from poor nutrition. They ate primarily ultraprocessed food because it was cheap and available in their communities.

We must address our national health calamity as soon as possible. The Covid-19 epidemic impacted Americans with chronic metabolic syndrome conditions most severely. We know that metabolic syndrome diseases are food-related and can be prevented or reversed by healthy nutrition. Before a metabolic syndrome disease develops into a clinical condition, we must take steps to avoid it. A caring nation's responsibility should be to prevent the disease in its people. Otherwise, we are sentencing those we are attempting to assist to a lifetime of misery. Our country must take steps to correct the issue of an unhealthy food environment. We must do this now because the human race experiencing another pandemic is inevitable.

§ § §

CHAPTER 09.

PRINCIPLES OF PERSONAL NATURAL NUTRITION

Food corporations' ultraprocessed meals, as well as their overwhelming advertising on public communication networks and social media, have led us to adopt incorrigible eating habits during the last 50 years. Although it may be difficult to resist their tempting food suggestions, remember that we don't have to fall for their propaganda. Because you have free will, you don't have to accept or be persuaded by such messages, which is why food companies spend so much money on advertising.

Many of you are already aware of some of these principles, but we want to provide a quick, easy and concise reference. We've also included a section on eating habits and routines derived from the positive outcomes of the Cuban health crisis that are supported by modern research. These guidelines are not intended for the thin and healthy. Those are the fortunate individuals who can eat almost anything without gaining weight and remain relatively healthy. However, those normal-weight individuals that eat ultraprocesseed food eventually developed insulin resistance and type 2 diabetes. In the United States, there are more normal-weight people with type 2 diabetes than obese people with the disease (see Appendix D.) The principles apply to the vast majority of people in this country who are overweight and suffer from chronic illnesses that impair their quality of life. If you fall into this category, most of the foods we advise you to avoid are processed foods high in carbohydrates and sugar, which raise insulin in our body and induce a hormonal imbalance, causing fat to accumulate in our cells.

We don't recommend any particular diet since we feel that any diet to be effective must be personalized to the individual. The majority of diets are based on the idea that food is the most crucial variable. According to new research, the most critical variable is the person, not the food, especially if you have an underlying health condition. Please read the nutritional labels on the packaging carefully. If it contains unhealthy ingredients or unpronounceable compounds or has more than 5 ingredients, do not eat it. We'll start with foods to avoid and then highlight foods you can eat if you're not allergic to them, finishing up with some suggestions for eating routines that you can try and light physical activities you can do a few times a week.

Foods to Avoid

- **Avoid ultraprocessed foods** from fast-food outlets, food trucks, restaurant chains, and any processed packaged food from the supermarket. Several new natural (real) food restaurants and food trucks with healthy meals are opening up that you might consider.

- **Avoid refined grains, including whole grains** such as bread, bagels, spaghetti, pancakes, waffles, muffins, cornbread, and cakes, to name a few.
- **Avoid gravy or other dressings** such as store-bought gravy or dressings. These products frequently contain sugar and other chemical substances that are not healthy for you.
- **Avoid sugar, foods containing sugar, all sweets, and sugary beverages**. Sugar has 252 different designations, as discussed in Chapter 3). Avoid pastries, cakes, sugary drinks, and fruit juices, which are high in fructose but low in fiber, and keep in mind that sugar is found in 80 percent of packaged foods on supermarkets shelves.
- **Avoid cooking with vegetable oils** since they contain high levels of omega-6 fats, and the oil extraction process is unhealthy. Mayonnaise, salad dressing, non-dairy butter, and margarine made with those oils are not to be consumed.
- **Avoid corn-fed meats, poultry, and farm fish.** Branched-chain amino acids are in high concentration

in corn products and are unhealthy unless you are a bodybuilder. Those foods usually contain antibiotics.

- **Avoid all packaged snacks** despite the marketing hype on their containers or the claims that they are low-calorie foods. They are not nutritious in cans, bottles, cartons, boxes, or frozen-food containers and are high on salt.

- **Avoid processed foods with salt.** Too much sodium has been linked to high blood pressure, which leads to a higher risk of heart disease, stroke, and kidney problems. The FDA advises limiting your salt intake to 2.3 grams (one U.S. teaspoon) per day. If you have hypertension (high blood pressure), your intake should be no more than 1.5 grams per day. If you eat processed foods or in fast food outlets, your food will exceed the FDA's recommendation after only one meal.

- **Avoid all human-made industrialized foods.** You should avoid human-made foods like margarine, refined food products from seeds to grains and sugar, and vegetable oils and sugary (sweet) drinks, including fruit juices that concentrate the fructose without the benefit of the fiber.

- **Avoid fortified (enriched) foods.** Many packaged processed foods are fortified with synthetic vitamins and minerals. For some people, these synthetic substances can be a problem; for instance, iron can cause insulin resistance.

- **Avoid fried foods when eating out.** Whether you eat at a fast-food outlet or a neighborhood restaurant, or a restaurant chain, avoid fried foods because almost all restaurants reuse vegetable oils for weeks, reheating them many times. Vegetable oils are hazardous for your health, especially when reheated.
- **Avoid foods to which you are allergic.** Some people are allergic to a particular food or a specific compound in food.

Foods Worth Eating

- **Do eat** natural nutritional meals to maintain good health. Again, we are not endorsing any particular diet but are providing you with some natural (real) and nutritious food principles.
- **Do eat** organic vegetables, especially green vegetables. If organic food is out of reach, non-organic vegetables are preferable to fast foods.
- **Do eat** dry legumes, such as beans. The drying process has not harmed the nutritional value of the bean.
- **Do eat** and cook with natural fats such as lard, dairy butter, and dairy ghee. If you must fry a food, use dairy

ghee: it has a high smoke point. Use extra virgin olive oil and avocado oil for your salad.

- **Do eat** eggs, poultry, and wild fish. They contain the amino acid tryptophan, a precursor of serotonin production, and serotonin, an essential brain neurotransmitter.
- **Do eat** starchy foods on occasion. If you wish to eat potatoes, boil them and butter them with dairy butter. Instead of ordinary rice, which may contain inorganic arsenic [5], eat cauliflower rice. The FDA has found that eating rice on a regular basis may increase the risk of lung and bladder cancer.[103] If you are prediabetic, avoid all starchy foods.
- **Do eat** meat from pasture-raised animals (beef, lamb, pork, chicken). Nonorganic meat from animals that aren't corn-fed or treated with antibiotics will suffice if you can't afford pasture-raised meats.

---

[5] The amount of arsenic in rice depends on the variety of rice and where it was grown. Brown rice absorbs more arsenic while growing than white, with basmati rice regularly having the lowest levels when tested. Regional differences matter too. Rice grown in Arkansas, Texas, Louisiana, and most other U.S. states had the highest inorganic arsenic levels. Inorganic arsenic is the kind that is dangerous and is associated with adverse health effects. The FDA has found inorganic arsenic in rice cause lung and bladder cancer when eating it in a regular basis.

- **Do eat** wild-caught fish, but stay away from farm fish, which are frequently treated with antibiotics and corn-fed.
- **Do drink** plenty of water throughout the day. Drink water slowly just until you are satiated.
- **Do not** overload helpings on your plate. You can serve yourself less food by using a smaller plate. Also, with each mouthful, eat slower and in smaller portions to give your stomach time to send a signal to your brain that you are full.
- **Do not** snack between meals, but if you cannot contain yourself, drink tea or coffee (without sugar); if you must snack, eat a raw vegetable, raw fruit, or raw unsalted nuts.

The circadian rhythm is an internal, natural process that regulates the sleep-wake cycle and occurs every 24 hours. It can refer to any process originating within an organism caused by factors within the body or mind or from internal structural or functional causes and responses to the environment. We recommend that you practice the following suggestions on a schedule or as regularly as you can during the day or week.

Eating Habits and Routines Worth Following

- **Eat** no more than three meals a day (breakfast, lunch, and dinner) and avoid snacking during the day.
- **Eat** your meals at the same time each day whenever feasible.
- **Eat** small portions and slowly, rather than rushing.
- **Do practice time-restricted feeding** and make it a habit. You might want to skip breakfast three or four times a week and eat only two meals in 8 hours (lunch and dinner). After a few weeks of practicing eating two meals per day, you may want to extend the time-restricted feeding to one meal a day (OMAD) a couple of times each week.
- **Do practice intermittent fasting** once a month or at least once a quarter if you can. If you are successful with the OMAD routine, you can increase it to 48 hours. We recommend that you check with a physician if you do 48 hours or more of fasting.
- **Do vary your meals** daily. Varying the type of food you eat to obtain different nutrients for your body is necessary even if you consume natural (real) foods.
- **Do physical activities** daily, such as walking or riding a bicycle, and relax before meals.

Upton Sinclair wrote about his experiences with nutrition and fasting in *The Fasting Cure*, published in 1911. He said, "In those [earlier] days, I believed something because other people told me; today, I know something different because I tried it upon myself."[99]

§ § §

CHAPTER 10.

A PUBLIC FOOD TRUST AUTHORITY (PFTA)

The Food and Drug Administration (FDA) is an agency "captured" by the food and pharmaceutical industries. The agency head is a political appointee of the U.S. President and usually has a background in one of the industries. The stated mission of the FDA is to protect the public health by ensuring the safety, efficacy, and security of human and veterinary drugs, biological products, and medical devices, and by ensuring the safety of our nation's food supply, cosmetics, and products that emit radiation.[104] There are just too many competing interests driving the agency in different ways. Unfortunately, the agency is moving away from having a more rigorous system for evaluating and approving slow-acting chronic toxic compounds that impact public health in the United States.

When a food manufacturer adds back nutrients that may have been removed during processing, they are fortifying the food. Milk is an example of a *food fortification* mandated by the government. During pasteurization and homogenization of milk, some vitamins are lost in the process. Thus, to comply with the regulations, the dairy industry is mandated to add vitamins A and D back into the milk. It would be best never to assume that adding a nutrient to a processed food will lead to the nutrient being absorbed and available to the body's cells. For example, skim milk is made by removing the fat from milk and adding in vitamins A and D. Both vitamins A and D are fat-soluble, not water-soluble. In other words, someone who does not consume fat with their milk will not obtain these vitamins as they would from whole milk, which contains fat. Also, the toxic properties of various other micronutrients regularly added to foods are a serious concern.

Another classification is *additives*, substances added to food to preserve flavor or improve its taste and appearance. A total of 19 different categories of food additives are available. The Food and Drug Administration (FDA) has approved the use of 3,000 food additives within that category. As a result, some products are labeled "generally recognized as safe" (GRAS). Even though the federal government has approved using some of these additives in our food supply, some food additives may still be harmful to our health. For this reason and others, it is preferable to purchase and consume natural food or food that has undergone a minimum amount of processing.

The GRAS lists, which the FDA is supposed to monitor, show chemical compounds that are currently used in foods. When a new chemical (additive) is added to the list, it is rarely removed. The FDA has never gone through the procedure of approving numerous food additives. According to Consumers Union scientists, many additives in our food supply are never tested because the GRAS designation is voluntary. Companies can choose to notify the FDA about their product instead of being required to register food additives. Adding a substance to the list creates significant conflicts of interest, and the FDA seldom reviews the compounds. This indifference suggests that the FDA does not place a high priority on public healthy food items.

The FDA-approved food additives are presumed "safe for human consumption," though this presumption may not always be correct. Food and color additives have been linked to allergic reactions and others to cancer, asthma, and congenital disabilities.[105] Foods that have been linked to heart disease, such as trans fats (vegetable oils), have been removed from the GRAS list after more than 50 years of heart disease mortality statistics. The FDA also requires that all ingredients be listed on a food label. Still, additives are frequently listed without specificity, like spices or flavoring. Thus, consumers do not know what they are eating. According to the Government Accountability Office (GAO), the FDA is not ensuring the safety of many chemicals. The consumer is constantly exposed to a chemical soup, the ingredients of which may interact to produce unanticipated health effects. Over 100 countries accept the FDA GRAS determinations of additives. It can become a global problem because those countries rely on the United States for the safety of the chemical ingredients they add to their food. The FDA does not have an unbiased and robust, safe scientific method to evaluate the long-term suitability of these chemicals to human biochemistry. As proof, we can ask, what has the FDA done in the last 50 years to prevent or inform the public about potentially hazardous food additives? Literally nothing. Otherwise, we would not be facing the current health crisis. It is up to us, the people, to prioritize our health.

Public Food Trust Authority: Framework

Despite our ideological belief in "government for the people," we know that other interests influence the federal government as its sometimes slow in acting on people's behalf. In Appendix C (*Government in the Public Interest?),* we cite cases where federal agencies have taken 12 to over 90 years to remedy a particular public health hazard. For more than 5 decades, our current national health crisis has been in the making. We're still waiting for the government to make sound recommendations to replace and revise the MyPlate nutritional guidelines and update the ingredients label with more meaningful information.

We sincerely believe that it is time for people to take charge of their own health. An *independent non-profit organization* is required to keep records on nutritious and edible foods as well as non-harmful substances in the food supply. We would call it the Public Food Trust Authority (PFTA). We recommend that some of the experts on our honor wall who have founded organizations in their fields of interest join the PFTA board of directors. The PFTA's first task would be to compile a list of food ingredients that have been proven to be healthy over time and are considered human-safe. Any other food additive not thoroughly tested will not be listed and considered not safe for human consumption. The nutrition facts labels should be improved to include what has been done to the food. The NOVA classification should be included as part of the nutritional facts. The organization's responsibilities would be expanded as needed.

To earn the public's trust rather than being just another well-intentioned organization, the board will have to define the PFTA mission, including the oversight of areas currently being disregarded by the FDA, such as slow (chronic) toxic substances. "Divided we fall; united we can influence policy and build public trust," as the modified proverb goes; it seems to apply. The PFTA board of directors will need biochemists, medical physicians, biochemistry-trained nutritionists, safe food consumer advocates, one member of the U.S. Senate and one member of the U.S. House of Representatives, and members of the general public.

Public Food Trust Authority: Mission, Beginnings

We need help in determining the organization's mission and outlining its responsibilities. OpenFoodFacts.org is a global website that lists the nutrients in packaged foods and ingredient labels. It's a place to start, but we need more than just information. The French have attempted to replace the ingredients label with something more meaningful: the Nutri-Score. Although far superior to the United States' labeling system, it was complex and vehemently opposed by the global food industry. Many Western European countries have voluntarily adopted Nutri-Score.[106] To be successful, the PFTA must advocate for a revised nutrition label, as described in Chapter 11.

The PFTA can support and expand objective randomized research on healthy or dangerous substances in the food supply and human nutrition. There are numerous ways for the organization to become a valued public asset and validate the healthiness of foods for consumers. One way would be to develop a smartphone application that identifies healthy and unhealthy ingredients in foods sold at fast-food outlets and restaurant chains. For each food product, we need to create a simple grading scale that indicates whether the food is:

(1) healthy (green)
(2) somewhat healthy (amber)
(3) somewhat unhealthy (blue) or
(4) extremely unhealthy (red).

It needs to be simple so consumers can understand it at a glance. The grading scale will match the NOVA group categories 1 through 4 (see Chapter 11.) This application will have to be tested before it is released to the public. If successful, the approach can be extended to packaged convenience food sold in supermarkets. The PFTA can work with private companies developing applications for healthy eating and tracking the effects of different foods on the individual to help build those applications database and bring them to the market.

The PFTA should be ready to administer and develop a massive general advertising campaign to be put in motion to change the public behavior of eating unhealthy food. The organization will need to consult with psychologists and sociologists on changing crowd behavior. The potential advertising campaign will be discussed in more detail in Chapter 11.

The database repository of the PFTA can be used to evaluate the compounds and activities of processed food products. This information will serve as input for the disvaluing assessment defined in Chapter 12. The calculation of the disvaluing evaluation will be labeled the *Edible Disvaluing Activity Levy* (EDAL).

The PFTA will need to work with academic institutions to develop natural nutrition standards for the public. The standards, at a minimum, should address age, gender, and health. People suffering from metabolic syndrome or other diseases will need a personalized diet based on their underlying conditions; further details are in Chapter 11.

The U.S. government cannot continue allowing major food companies to introduce chemicals into the food supply and profit from doing so for 50 or 100 years while people suffer from their chemicals. We need legislation to set up a rigorous review process for new substances being introduced into the food supply that the FDA can and has the expertise to administer. The process should have the same stringent criteria as the process for introducing a new drug to the public. Only if a substance is scientifically proved to be beneficial should a food company be allowed to introduce it into the food supply. The food companies should not be allowed to add chemicals into the food supply to make food look more appealing and palatable; see Chapter 11 for more details.

The PFTA needs to take on this initiative, become a health advocate for the nation, and lobby the U.S. Congress when necessary. We can no longer sit on the sidelines.

§ § §

CHAPTER 11.

NATIONAL NUTRITIONAL HEALTH: A STRATEGY

The novelist and essayist Marcel Proust once wrote, "The real voyage of discovery consists not in seeking new landscapes, but in having new eyes." Our current healthcare model of treating individuals when they become ill is incredibly expensive for the country. Eventually, it will lead to healthcare rationing. Having a strategy to keep individuals from becoming sick is crucial for preventing an unhealthy population. Therefore, this chapter will be devoted to developing and recommending a strategy for dealing with our country's health crisis.

We follow that Marcel Proust maxim in presenting a natural nutritional intervention for our unhealthy food environment. It has been there all along; it just needs to be looked at from a different perspective. In old photos from the 1950s and 1960s, we see people walking along a street or in a school graduation procession or grandparents posing for a family picture. The striking feature of those photos is that almost everyone is thin; seldom do you see an overweight person.

What major event happened in this country in the 1970s that caused the population in the 1980s to gain weight at an alarming rate? The publication in 1977 of the *Dietary Goals for the United States* and in 1980 of *Nutrition and Your Health: Dietary Guidelines for Americans* was drawn up by the Senate Select Committee on Nutrition and Human Needs. The guidelines, unfortunately, led to the promotion of low-fat/high-carb diets. Criticisms of the guidelines and dietary approach have since led to several revisions, but they are still surrounded by controversy. The guidelines have directly contributed to the problem by advocating a low-fat/high-carb diet and indirectly urging the food industry to produce more low-fat/high carb goods, resulting in an overabundance of factory-made ultraprocessed food.

Most of the current healthcare costs (75 percent) are associated with chronic metabolic syndrome diseases. Type 2 diabetes is the sentinel disease of metabolic syndrome.[29] Appendix D demonstrates that type 2 diabetes is a food-related and lifestyle disease that can be treated, reversed, and cured with the appropriate personalized natural (real) food diet. The Cuban health crisis experience has shown that we can reverse metabolic syndrome diseases at a national level by changing our diet. The changes can substantially reduce healthcare costs.

Without a doubt, our current food environment has degraded our quality of life and is slowly killing us. New food chemical compounds are being introduced at a rapid pace by the food and chemical sectors. Companies attempt to differentiate their food items by developing chemicals and adding them to the food supply. They do not seek to provide nutritional food; rather, the degree of processing is important in producing palatable flavors, appealing appearance, and chewable texture with addictive substances. They have not proved any benefit to the consumer, justified the need for such components, or addressed how the new compounds interact with existing chemical substances and the long-term consequences on human physiology. They've had a free ride experimenting with human health in real-time, resulting in the current health catastrophe in the United States and other countries. As a result, food manufacturers must discontinue the use of harmful chemical components in their processed foods. Because they are unlikely to change their ways voluntarily, we proposed the following national strategy, resulting in significant improvements in these seven areas.

1. A massive public education campaign on nutrition and natural foods to change the current unhealthy eating behaviors
2. A mechanism to reduce the current level of consumption of processed and ultraprocessed foods
3. Tax incentives for food companies to produce healthy convenience foods
4. A robust testing procedure for introducing new chemical ingredients, their health benefits, and nutritional justification before they are included in the GRAS list
5. The United States needs a new ingredients label that better describe the ingredients and the level of processing of the food

6. The training of nutritionists and the education of dietitians and primary physicians on the nutritional biochemistry of natural foods
7. Personalized nutrition plans for people with metabolic syndrome diseases and the updating of 21st-century dietary practices

Item 1. A massive public education campaign on nutrition and natural foods to change the current unhealthy eating behaviors

Whether we like it or not, our country needs a strategy that explains what makes a healthy and nutritional diet. We are not talking about that small percentage of the population that understands that eating natural and healthy foods is essential and practices that way of eating. We are referring to the general public who still believe that our government and health institutions protect their health interests and safeguard our food supply from unhealthy products, even though harmful products are abundantly available. The public has given credence to those institutions based on press releases about their involvement when food-borne bacterial illnesses creep into the food supply, such as *Salmonella* and *Escherichia coli* infections. These news stories tend to reinforce the belief that the FDA monitors the food supply for the general public. Although this may be true in the reported situations, it is not true of the foods that cause chronic diseases. This gap in policy needs to be addressed.

The public is constantly bombarded with food company advertising that is misleading and detrimental to their health. The advertising is for industrialized ultraprocessed convenience foods packaged and sold on grocery shelves, freezers, fast-food outlets, and restaurant chains. Our food supply has become unhealthy over the last 50 years with the introduction of more and more ultraprocessed foods by the food industry. The explosion in unhealthy foods was prompted by the dietary goals of the Senate Select Committee on Nutrition and Human Needs of 1977, led by the late U.S. Senator George McGovern. Although the goals and guidelines were well-intentioned, they indirectly provided the means for the food companies to ramp up their industrial food processing methods and start the obesity and diabetes epidemic. If you need proof, as we said before, all you have to do is look at photos of people walking on the streets of any city before the 1960s. You will see that the majority were normal-weight people; very rarely do you see an obese individual as you do in today's photos.

In the last 50 years, the two-income household has become the norm. Processed convenience foods have also become the norm in the home. To learn how to prepare our foods, we depend on TV cooking programs, cooking YouTube channels, and internet social media sponsored by food corporations. When we allow corporations to take on traditional family roles, we find that corporations do not have our best interests in mind. They care about selling their ultraprocessed convenience foods and staying ahead of the competition; they are not concerned about our health. They've created an unhealthy food environment that's only growing worse. It must end, but the food and chemical industries have the upper hand because of the vast sums of money they can spend on advertising their unhealthy processed food products and lobbyist to influence regulators. The U.S. government does not have the will or incentive to regulate food companies. We need to rebalance the scales and start teaching the country how to eat healthy again. Although we no longer have time to cook, small entrepreneurs are producing convenience nutritional foods free of harmful chemicals. Food companies are not on the people's side. The corporations are attempting to attract you to buy their products by concealing hazardous food ingredients and deceiving you, the consumer, through misleading advertising.

We must overcome chronic metabolic syndrome diseases in our population. We must educate the public about what constitutes unhealthy food and healthy natural food and identify food products that are minimally processed. To accomplish this, we will need a massive advertising campaign to counter the one used by the food industry to promote their ultraprocessed unhealthy foods. Unfortunately, food companies have influenced government agencies for more than 50 years, becoming more pervasive today. If government agencies attempt to educate the public about the benefits of eating natural foods, food corporations will accuse the government of establishing a nanny state. We propose that the

Public Food Trust Authority, as described in Chapter 10, manage the campaign and serve as a national educator and remain an independent organization.

The campaign should be massive and communicated on all the media networks, such as social media, blogs, and gaming channels on the Internet; in newspapers and magazines; in school curriculums; on billboards; and (significantly) as part of children's programming on TV and in K through 12-grade schools. The campaign should last for at least 5 years or until the food companies change their unhealthy foods and stop adding damaging chemicals to their foods. In our democracy, it is the only way to level the playing field without regulation or infringing on the people's right to choose. How is the U.S. government going to fund that campaign?

Item 2. A mechanism to reduce the current level of consumption of processed and ultraprocessed foods

The government will not be able to legislate unhealthy ultraprocessed foods out of the food supply. Most people will oppose this even though it is for their benefit. The food companies will try to influence legislators by giving them political donations and using an advertising campaign to confuse the public on the merit of the issues. They will use the "freedom of choice" slogan again as they have done in the states where attempts were made to limit the supersizing of beverages sold at certain food outlets. We need an advertising countercampaign that promotes healthy variants to re-educate the people.

We have a government tool, taxation, to make it more difficult for food companies to influence legislation. Still, in order for the U.S. Congress to introduce a new method of taxation, it needs a public rationale for doing so.

Rationale. When an industry produces unhealthy products, as has been the case with the food industry for over 50 years, it is time for the government to take action. Food companies, instead of rethinking their behavior and making changes, their leaders have hastened to push unhealthy processed food products onto the market. The FDA does not consider their goods hazardous (toxic) because they do not kill (poison) you immediately. Still, they are far worse since they make you sick, cause you to suffer for years, degrade your quality of life, and ultimately cause you to die prematurely.

Dietary risk factors are the leading causes of mortality and disability globally; dietary risks were estimated to account for 10.3 million deaths worldwide in 2016. Therefore, curbing the adverse effects of an unhealthy diet is a significant challenge in public health.[107] It is long overdue for our government to impose a tax on harmful food products and utilize the proceeds to educate the public and recoup the healthcare expenditures for the harm of those diseases.

Taxation. Although we are opposed to new taxes, we realized that the U.S. Congress might have no alternative but to assess new taxes to handle the level of metabolic syndrome in our country. The government needs to be more creative when introducing and levying the tax. The tax should be on the food companies' revenue from processed food items that are the most profitable products of food companies. There will be no taxes on natural food.

1. The tax will be on the food companies' revenue derived from processed and ultraprocessed food items categorized as a 3 or 4 under the NOVA classification. The companies may raise prices to recover the tax, but it will be detrimental to their sales.

2. The right of consumers to make their own decisions will not be infringed upon.

3. The government should fund a public awareness campaign to educate consumers on buying and eating healthy foods from this tax revenue assessment.

4. Finally, the food companies can reduce the tax burden by eliminating the hazardous compounds in processed food and producing healthier food.

In this modern era, whoever has the money to control the means of communication controls the agenda. When that control is detrimental to the public good, it must be curtailed. If they cannot be curtailed through regulation or because of constitutional issues, then they must be balanced. Chapter 12 will introduce a new tax concept to allow the government to attain those objectives and balance consumer and food companies' messages.

Item 3. Tax incentives for food companies to produce healthy convenience foods

Our aim is not to criticize food companies but to draw their attention to how their behavior and the products they release into the market are harming people. An executive can alter a company's behavior by introducing healthy and nutritional food products that are free of all unhealthy chemicals. In the coming years, the country will require your management expertise and food competence. Every 10 years, the population of the United States increases by 20 million people. In another 50 years, the nation will be home to an additional 100 million people who need healthy food. The government and the country's economy cannot afford the healthcare costs and productivity loss of allowing your companies to produce the quantity of ultraprocessed meals currently being manufactured. Continue to make and promote harmful ultraprocessed foods, and the United States will soon cease to be a viable nation because it will be a nation of sick people.

As an incentive to make healthier food, the disvaluing levy (tax) will decrease as food companies reduce their unhealthy ingredients in a food product. If the number of harmful chemicals added falls to zero, a levy would no longer be assessed on that food item. The food executives know how to make healthy food without using dangerous chemicals; they have done this in the past. New entrepreneurs are introducing nutritious and healthy food products to the market. Why can't you?

Item 4. A robust testing procedure for introducing new chemical ingredients, their health benefits, and nutritional justification before they are included in the GRAS list

The FDA needs to establish a more robust procedure than the one currently employed to introduce substances into the food supply. Furthermore, the firm or individual that created the chemical should explain the ingredient's health benefits and justify the need for such a chemical in food products. If the new ingredient does not provide any additional benefits beyond existing components, it should not be approved.

Some aspects of the review of new drugs by the FDA's Center for Drug Evaluation and Research (CDER) may help. The CDER is a sciencc-led body in charge of reviewing a drug before it is produced for sale. The CDER reviewers are an independent team of clinicians and scientists who carefully assess a new drug's safety, efficacy, and labeling. Following approval, the FDA monitors pharmaceuticals as they become available to ensure they remain safe and effective.

Substances added to food are frequently subjected to a review that may allow their inclusion on the Generally Recognized as Safe (GRAS) list. The process and significance of granting the GRAS label to a food ingredient differ from the FDA approval process of a new drug. The FDA initially created the GRAS designation to apply to commonly available ingredients such as vinegar and baking soda. The list of substances eventually grew so long that the FDA began to allow voluntary additions to the GRAS list without formal approval. It resulted in the acceptance of chemicals, substances, or ingredients deemed safe by food industry scientists. Food additives are now subject to much less scrutiny than FDA-approved additives in the past and are subject to the biases of food industry scientists. Most people are unaware of this and believe that the FDA has reviewed GRAS additives.

The label given in both the CDER and GRAS processes is permanently restricted to the drug's or additive's intended circumstances of use. The CDER and GRAS processes, on the other hand, are based on different levels of access to scientific data and information and involve different types of reviews. The CDER process is far more stringent and extensive. Although scientific data and information about a substance are supposed to be widely available in order to obtain a GRAS label, and competent experts are supposed to agree that the data and information establish that the substance is safe under the conditions of its intended use, the approval process is uneven, not always scientific, and can be influenced by corporate interests. In other words, the GRAS process is ineffective and has little or no involvement from the FDA. Some efforts have been made in the last ten years to improve the rigor of the process, but it remains insufficient, and many believe it should be replaced.

If this country wants to make some inroads into the safety of processed food, then this significant regulatory gap needs to be addressed. It is a Congressional issue that must be corrected. If the U.S. Congress is unwilling to make new regulations to make the process as robust as the introduction of new drugs, then the PFTA should take the initiative to list the additives that are deemed safe.

Item 5. The United States needs a new nutrition label that better describe the ingredients and the level of processing of the food

In the United States, we need new nutritional labeling for food ingredients. New labeling can provide strong incentives to the food industry to reformulate its products, improve their nutritional quality, and eliminate hazardous food chemicals.[106] According to the NOVA classification (see Appendix B), food processing involves physical, biological, and chemical processes that occur after foods are taken from nature and before they are cooked and consumed or used to prepare other food products and meals. The NOVA classification states that controlling food processing, rather than examining nutrients, should be foremost in shaping nutritional policy. The key topic that the FDA should investigate is processed food labeling, and NOVA is the best tool that has been designed thus far.[108]

We need to figure out which elements and compounds, such as processed foods, harmful ingredients, and slow-acting chronic toxins cause long-term harm to humans. The NOVA classification, which categorizes the various degrees of food processing, can better determine the potential for toxic compounds than the Nutrition Facts label in the United States today. The NOVA classification contains four categories:

Group 1. Unprocessed or minimally processed foods
Group 2. Processed culinary ingredients
Group 3. Processed foods
Group 4. Ultraprocessed food and drink products

We should also consider adding color code to those groups:

group 1, **green** to indicate it is healthy to eat
group 2, **amber** to indicate it is somewhat healthy to eat
group 3, **blue** to indicate it is somewhat unhealthy to eat
group 4, **red** to indicate it is extremely unhealthy to eat

The nutrition label should include the metabolic function of the food we are consuming. For example, let us take sugar which is made of sucrose, a nutrient. Sucrose is made of 2 compounds, glucose 50 percent, and fructose also 50 percent. The glucose is metabolized in the muscle and cells, while the fructose is metabolized in the liver. The nutrition facts label should read:

- Total Carb.: 8 grams – daily value (% DV) is 4 percent
    - Sugar: 8 grams
        - Glucose: 4 grams – metabolized in muscle & cells
        - Fructose: 4 grams – metabolized in the liver

Another thing the label should include is a consistent serving size. The industry persuaded the FDA to adopt an unrealistic serving size on the nutrition facts label. For example, the nutrition facts on a bottle of ketchup are as follows:

- Serving size: Tablespoon (17 grams),
- Calories: 20,
- Sodium: 160 milligrams – daily value (% DV) is 7 percent
- Total Carb.: 5 grams – daily value (% DV) is 2 percent
    - Sugar: 4 grams

The serving size of one tablespoon for ketchup is highly deceptive, and the business does it on purpose. If we use a more realistic serving size of 2 tablespoons or 34 grams, the numbers are as follows:

- Serving size: 2 Tablespoon (34 grams),
- Calories: 40,
- Sodium: 320 milligrams – daily value (% DV) is 14 percent
- Total Carb.: 10 grams – daily value (% DV) is 4 percent
    - Sugar: 8 grams

Suddenly, you realize that 2 tablespoons include 40 calories, 320 milligrams of sodium, and 8 grams of sugar, which is one-third

(33%) of the American Heart Association's recommended daily intake for sugar.

Trans fats are a type of fat primarily found in fast food and processed meals of all types and are known to be harmful to your health. Trans fats, often known as "partially hydrogenated oils," are used to keep foods from melting at room temperature and keep them fresher for longer. According to FDA regulations, less than half a gram (.5) of trans fat is not required to be recorded on the nutrition facts label. When you read the words "trans fat zero percent," that may imply you can have .4 grams of trans fat per tablespoon, and the manufacturer does not have to state the amount. Realistically, cooking with vegetable oil needs 2 to 4 teaspoons, so your actual trans fat consumption ranges from.8 to 1.6 grams. If you fry your food, it requires at least a cup of vegetable oil, which contains 19 grams of trans fat, and trans fat has been proven to cause heart disease, inflammation, higher "bad" LDL cholesterol, and lower "good" HDL cholesterol levels. It raises your chance of heart disease and stroke, as well as high blood pressure and obesity, increases your risk of type 2 diabetes, Alzheimer's disease, and some forms of cancer and other diseases. Remember, "0" percent trans fat does not mean zero; it means it is less than .5 percent.

As discussed in the previous chapter, the French tried to replace the nutrition label with more meaningful data: the Nutri-Score. Although considerably superior to the labeling system in the United States, it was complicated and vigorously opposed by the global food industry. Nutri-Score was voluntarily adopted by several

Western European nations, although not all food companies have complied.[106]

Item 6. The training of nutritionists and the education of dietitians and primary physicians on the nutritional biochemistry of natural foods

It should be evident from the current health calamity that the dietary advice that dietitians and physicians have been giving to patients and the public for the last 50 years is not working. The dietary suggestions they recommend are based on governmental dietary guidelines. Although this is safe for physicians and dietitians, it does not help patients with diabetes or obesity. Although change is slow, many physicians and dietitians are beginning to question what they were taught about calories and nutrition.

A calorie is a unit of measurement in physics. Our bodies are incapable of calculating calories. Food is metabolized by our bodies to produce energy, and different foods metabolize differently. Sugar is an example of a carbohydrate made up of equal parts glucose and sucrose. A 180-pound person consumes an 8-ounce glass of orange juice, containing 110 calories, 102 of which are sugar (26 grams). One-half of the 102 calories or 51 glucose calories are metabolized by 175 pounds of cells and muscles. A 5-pound liver metabolizes the other half of the 51 fructose calories. The fructose (sugar) level eventually overwhelms the liver's ability to metabolize it, resulting in fatty liver and insulin resistance. If those calories had come from green vegetables or meat, the entire body would have metabolized them. As a result, a calorie is not a calorie because they are metabolized differently. Nutritional biochemistry training is needed to understand how the human body metabolizes different foods. Understanding the intestinal microbiome and its role in human biochemistry is also critical. In the twenty-first century, the human diet will be dependent on biochemistry, and physicians and dietitians will need to update their training.

Biochemists are researching compounds in natural foods that help prevent and reverse diseases. For example, Theodore Fotsis, a Greek scientist, released a seminal paper in 1993. He revealed that the urine of healthy Japanese men and women who ate soy foods contained genistein, a natural chemical with potent anti-cancer properties. Dr. Fotsis found in laboratory studies that genistein reduced the number of tumor-induced blood vessels. Genistein was later demonstrated to directly inhibit the growth of four different types of cancer cells.[109] Because the body does not produce genistein, its only source is edible plants.[110] According to Dr. William Li, more than 100 foods, including soy, tomatoes, black raspberries, and pomegranates, can improve your body's ability to starve cancer cells and keep tumors small and harmless. Another example of biochemical research is Dr. Robert Lustig's study of sugar (fructose) in children. He was able to show that stopping the consumption of sugar in children for 10 days reversed a fatty liver to a normal healthy liver.[111]

Item 7. Personalized nutrition plans for people with metabolic syndrome diseases and the updating of 21st-century dietary practices

A nutritionist must consider that each person is physiologically distinctive and that different foods elicit diverse metabolic and hormonal responses. One person gains weight by eating a specific food; another person does not.[9] If the patient needs dietary intervention, we have to tailor the diet to advise and coach the patient using technological means. We need to use tools such as those outlined in the article *Personalized Nutrition by Prediction of Glycemic Responses.* [6][90]

The patient is counseled on which foods are natural (real) foods, why they are beneficial, and how they improve health. The patient is shown how hazardous foods, such as ultraprocessed foods, vegetable oils, sugary drinks, and snacks, have a detrimental impact on health. The patient needs to understand how often to eat and the importance of only eating three meals per day. For some patients, time-restricted feeding may be beneficial. Patients with health conditions require a personalized nutritional plan tailored to their

---

[6] Researchers at the Weizmann Institute of Science in Israel have developed an algorithm to measure the effects of different food types on a person's glucose levels and any spike in the levels produced by specific foods. They have found that people eating identical foods may have different glucose level responses. Their algorithm allows them to prescribe the best individualized diet for each patient to prevent the glucose spikes that are so dangerous with diabetes. See reference 90. Zeevi, D., et al., *Personalized nutrition by prediction of glycemic responses.* Cell, 2015. **Cell 163, 1079–1094**.

diseases, allergies, and other considerations such as gender and age. The term *personalized* is fundamental because the physiology of each person is different. In a personalized diet, the **person is the variable.** A particular food may be the right one for one person but may not suit another person.

The U.S. dietary goals were created for adult males in 1977. The formal guidelines have changed little over the years despite the fact that metabolic syndrome diseases have become rampant since the guidelines were first issued. It is time that the guidelines be modified to include the diversity of our population. Here are some suggestions for age-related cohorts' nutritional needs:

Infancy and Childhood

Group	Age
Newborn	0-1 month
Infant	2-23 months
Early childhood	2-7 years
Middle childhood	8-11 years
Adolescence/puberty*	12-19 years

*The age at puberty may vary by individual. Pregnant adolescents may have different dietary requirements than other adolescents.

Infancy and childhood are the most vital stages to focus on reversing obesity in children. These are the times to create healthy eating habits, especially in newborns. The food industry adds sugar to baby food to make it more palatable, but this causes newborns to become addicted to sugar. In addition, food companies often sponsor children's television programs and advertise unhealthy sugary foods.

Dr. Lustig's research on obese children has demonstrated that eliminating refined sugar from the diet can reverse a child's fatty liver in 10 days.[111] In his book *Food Fight*, Kelly Brownell stated that children need protection from an out-of-control food and advertising environment.[112]

Adulthood

Group	Age
Early adulthood*	20-55 years
Late adulthood	56-70 years
Senior adulthood	71+ years

*Pregnancy can occur at these ages, and the dietary requirements will be different.

Persons in early adulthood can lower their weight and keep it off. We know from research that once a person becomes obese after that stage in life, it is difficult to lose weight and keep it off.[113] The most successful diet for maintaining a healthy weight is a combination of natural (real) food and time-restricted feeding. Research has shown that when vegetable oils and refined sugars are significantly reduced or eliminated from the diet, there is a decrease in fatty liver incidence, reduced insulin resistance, and weight loss.[46, 75] There are no dietary guidelines for the age-related cohorts above. We recommend that the Public Food Trust Authority sponsor appropriate nutritional standards with universities' biochemical human nutrition departments. It is up to the American people to push for this strategy and have their congressperson support it.

§ § §

CHAPTER 12.

THE ECONOMIC CONCEPT OF DISVALUING: FUNDING A NATIONAL NUTRITIONAL STRATEGY

Our country's sick population with chronic metabolic syndrome diseases is growing, and unless we make substantial health changes, the government will be forced to ration healthcare. We cannot sustain a healthcare expenditure growing exponentially while the economy grows at 2 or 3 percent annually. As previously stated, the diseases afflicting the people of this country are food-related, specifically processed food. We know that the food industry can change to benefit the people, their consumers. They must do so either willingly or by taxation. The Cuban Crisis demonstrated how, in times of hardship, positive health benefits might be accomplished. We must take this difficult step for future generations to have long and healthy lives.

We developed the economic concept of *disvaluing* based in part on a publication by Credit Suisse Research, "Sugar Consumption at a Crossroads." It stated,

> "Regulators and health officials around the world have done little to address the impact of excess sugar consumption. We believe [***higher taxation on 'sugary' food and drinks***]

would be the best option to reduce sugar intake and [***help fund the fast-growing healthcare costs associated with diabetes type II and obesity***]. Economists generally agree that government intervention, including [***taxation, is justified when the market fails to provide the optimum amount of a good for society's well-being***]."[114]

The statement comes from a bank. If bankers can see clearly, why can't our government? How much longer must we wait for the government to act? We will assist them. Below is a proposal for them to act on to help the people of our country.

The Concept of Disvaluing: A New Health Policy

The tax option is a less appealing option for all parties involved. We loathe paying more taxes and giving the government authority over how they are spent, just like any other American. However, if the food companies do not change their market behavior of introducing more harmful products, taxes are the last choice for aiding our country. If a tax solution is required, we can be quite creative in developing that tax. We propose the notion of *disvaluing* as a new economic concept for corporate taxation. Before we go over the concept of disvaluing, let's go over the opposite of the concept: value-added.

"Value-added" can refer to measurements in economics, business finance, marketing, and accounting. In economics, it is the difference between overall sales within an industry and total costs of materials and services purchased from other firms over a certain period. The contribution of one industry sector to a country's GDP (gross domestic product) is known as economic value-added.

We should be familiar with the value-added concept in business marketing. A value-added situation occurs when a business adds enhancements such as functionality, services, or warranties to a product's value. When customers are willing to pay more for an enhancement, it is classified as a value-added improvement. Value-added is a competitive advantage gained by differentiating a product or service from that of a competitor. In other words, value-added is the difference between the price and the cost of a product. Thus, a value-added is a monetary phrase for an economic aspect that may be materially expressed and assessed. In some countries, although not in the United States, a value-added tax is assessed on a product. A value-added tax is a consumption tax levied on a product at each stage along the supply chain, from manufacturing to final purchase by the consumer. It is considered a regressive tax because it taxes consumption regardless of income.

We need a new way of looking at and measuring what's happening on with our country's wealth and people's health. When an industry negatively influences a country's GDP, the consequences need to be addressed; this is the case with the processed food industry and its products' impact on many aspects of our lives. Healthcare expenditures are increasing, labor productivity is declining, more and more assets are being used for treating sickness, and people suffer from an unhealthy food environment. The damages caused by processed foods surpass any possible contributions the processed foods might make to GDP.

Disvaluing, which captures reductions in value, is the opposite of value-added. Is disvaluing like depreciation, in which a building loses its original value over time? Not really; depreciation is planned obsolescence that occurs as the building ages. The disvaluing concept applies when production factors do not positively contribute to the nation's wealth. Initially, the production of such a product may appear to contribute to the economy, but with further analysis, it becomes evident that the product costs the country more than it contributes.

The disvaluing tax is not a regressive tax. It does not tax the added value of a product, which is a positive force in our economy. Still, it taxes the hazardous compounds and activities that harm consumers and negatively impacts our economy (see Chapter 13). The disvaluing tax is a targeted tax designed to address the unhealthy food environment caused by some processed food products produced by the food industry. As explained in Chapter 05, it corrects imbalances in our free-market economy. Corporations must be competitive to survive, but sometimes they cannot control the harm they cause to individuals and our economy. The pressure to outperform competitors can lead to aberrant behavior in an industry. Corporations produce harmful products and cannot stop doing so. At that point, an economic instrument is required to control disruptive behavior. When a government fails to intervene with meaningful legislation to correct an industry's negative behavior, the only tool left is taxation.

That was the message of Credit Suisse Bank when it justified a sugar tax. The tax cannot be regressive, as the value-added tax. It must be a tax targeted at repairing the damage caused by unhealthy processed food industry products. The disvaluing levy is the solution to this economic situation. To distinguish it from a value-added tax, we call it a levy rather than a tax.

A food manufacturer disvalues food when it takes natural food and degrades its matrix into a consumer product that is no longer natural. When the food industry introduces ingredients and chemicals that do not naturally occur in a food product, it disvalues the natural product nutrition; it creates a synthetic food matrix that does not benefit consumers but harms them over time. The value of food to the industry is determined not by whether it is beneficial or contains the necessary nutrients but by whether it can be sold as a palatable product with a long shelf life. Manufacturers value food products based on their type, degree, and purpose of processing to earn a profit. The manufacturer values those food attributes because they are the source of their revenue, and this is the specific area that will be taxed.

In macroeconomics, a standard partial productivity measure is labor productivity. *Labor productivity* is an indicator of economic growth, competitiveness, and living standards. The indicator helps explain economic growth, national wealth, and social development.

It is one area of the financial status of our country that is being undermined by the processed food industry. Almost half of our adult population suffers from chronic metabolic syndrome diseases. The illnesses continue to increase, impacting labor productivity and becoming a significant threat to our way of life and our country's future wealth (see Chapter 13.)

We must decide whether to allow the food companies to continue their reckless introduction of unhealthy processed food products into the market. It seems clear that stopping this behavior is essential. Therefore, we need to find a way to make companies end their harmful practices. Many state legislatures have tried to pass legislation to stop them, but their approach has failed. Therefore, it seems that the only viable option is to tax them.

The strategy for levying a disvaluing tax is twofold:

(1) It will encourage companies to change detrimental practices and become part of a healthy food environment

(2) Companies will be penalized, with a tax, if they do not change their harmful processed food practices.

Let us first explain how the levy will be calculated. The calculation must consider the artificial ingredients or compounds added to a processed food product, as well as the activities carried out to incorporate those ingredients and compounds into the food product. Vegetable oils, for example, are extracted from seeds or grains. Because chemical compounds are used to extract the oil from the seed or grain, each chemical is assigned a disvalue percentage.

Activities are carried out to extract the oil with a chemical, usually hexane, and remove it from the product, making it edible. Each of these activities is also assigned a disvalue percentage. The addition of disvalue percentages for chemical compounds and activities during the manufacturing process results in the levy percentage that will be applied to the revenue of food companies for vegetable oil products. The rates for the ingredients or compounds, as well as the activities, will be defined by the PFTA organization. The PFTA will calculate the disvaluing percentage of a product, in this case, vegetable oil. The calculation elements are as follows:

- Chemicals disvalue percent **X** cost of chemicals = chemicals levy amount
- Activities disvalue percent **X** cost of manufacturing activities = activities levy amount
- **(**chemicals levy amount + activities levy amount**)** / total cost of manufacturing = disvalue levy percent
- Vegetable oil revenue **X** disvalue levy percent = disvalue levy assessment

In step (1), the Public Food Trust Authority (PFTA) will be participating. The PFTA will educate the public through advertising and an internet website. The website will keep physicians and dietitians informed about nutrition biochemistry developments. Part of the PFTA mission will assist those affected by processed foods and connect them with qualified dietitians in their community. The levy on firms' processed foods revenue will help to support those activities. As processed food companies become subject to the levy, the PFTA will provide them with the opportunity to transition away from ultraprocessed goods and toward healthier food alternatives. The tax on processed foods will be reduced if the manufacturer retains the product's natural nutrition components while lowering or removing detrimental and synthetic additives.

Step (2) will increase the levy if the food manufacturer does not make the food product healthier. The aim would be to use the levy as leverage to make harmful ultraprocessed foods uneconomical for the food companies to produce. The levy will generate enough revenue to fund the national nutritional campaign for the next five years. Any additional annual revenue will go to lower healthcare costs. For example, if the levy collected in a fiscal year is $100 and the PFTA uses $20, the remaining $80 can be applied to healthcare costs. We hope that after 5 years, companies will be more focused on positive efforts to make food healthy, even if this means that the amount of taxes collected for disvaluing will be lower. It is likely that some amount will continue to be collected, and that amount could be used to keep the healthy food campaign ongoing, pay for the PFTA's administrative costs, and reduce healthcare costs. The PFTA will be reduced in size as the population becomes healthier and food nutrition quality improves.

As we explain in Chapter 11, the disvaluing levy should have the following objectives.

1. The tax will be on the food companies' revenue derived from processed and ultraprocessed food items categorized as a 3 or 4 under the NOVA classification. The companies may raise prices to recover the tax, but it will be detrimental to their sales.

2. The right of consumers to make their own decisions will not be infringed upon.

3. The government should fund a public awareness campaign to educate consumers on buying and eating healthy foods from this tax revenue assessment.

4. Finally, the food companies can reduce the tax burden by eliminating the hazardous compounds in processed food and producing healthier food.

The levy will be uniform throughout the country and avoid the cigarette sales tax issues that created interstate contraband. The states will continue to have the capability to add a sales tax to processed food. The independent non-profit PFTA will compile and publish a classification of unhealthy ingredients that will be used to calculate the disvaluing levy.

We understand that we may have to give up some control to the government to receive funding for the PFTA. However, if Congress is to have the nation's health as a priority, then the PFTA organization must be independent. The Department of Health and Human Services and its FDA are being pushed in too many different directions. They have neglected to meet their obligations to safeguard people from chronic diseases and to promote healthy living. Our current health crisis is proof of their lack of action. The U.S. Congress should take on some of this responsibility and also elect the managing director of the PFTA board of directors. Also, they should be selecting two of its members, one from the Senate and one from the House of Representatives, to be honorary members of the PFTA board of directors.

Federal Levy and Local Sales Tax: Disvaluing Funding

The disvaluing strategy is different than strategies for other taxes. Sales taxes, for instance, are generally applied to the final value (price) of a product. The disvaluing tax is assessed all along the path of production. It is calculated for each added chemical in a product and each harmful manufacturing process or other activity at each production stage and preparation until sold to the end consumer.

The levy percent will be assessed on the revenue produced by the sales of the processed food products. If the food company raises prices, it will impact the sales of its products.

We do not call it a tax but a levy; it sounds less burdensome and is differentiated from the value-added tax. Its full name is the ***Edible Disvaluing Activity Levy*** (EDAL). Let us explain it.

- **Edible** refers to the nature of a product, which is food consumed by humans.
- **Disvaluing** means that a product's nutritional value has decreased because its manufacturer has changed its original natural components to a non-natural food matrix, detrimental to human health.
- **Activity** refers to the steps taken to disvalue a food, such as grinding, washing, bleaching, adding chemicals, and disposing of the residual chemicals. The activities refer to the type, degree, and purpose of processing creating the non-natural food matrix.
- **Levy,** of course, is the imposition or collection of an assessment by the government.

The levy will be assessed on each manufacturing activity process, and ingredients added that disvalue a food. Based on the activities and ingredients used to create an ultraprocessed, chocolate creamy-wafer cookie, we can use the ingredients and activities and calculate the levy. For example, there are 15 ingredients added and 17 activities used to process the chocolate creamy-wafer. The result is a levy of 15 percent on the company's revenue for this cookie product.

As previously stated, a value-added tax is a tax levied at each stage of a supply chain. Our disvaluing tax differs from the value-added tax in that there is no additional tax imposed if there is no further disvaluation in the supply chain. The disvaluing tax (EDAL) was calculated at 15 percent in the case of the chocolate creamy-wafer. The rest of the supply chain is not doing anything to disvalue the product (wholesaler, distributor, retail outlet), so the EDAL is not calculated for any of their activities. In this case, the EDAL is only assessed, 15 percent, on the manufacturer revenue for chocolate creamy-wafers.

If we look at the example of raw sugar, the EDAL is 15 percent of the manufacturer revenue for raw sugar, but other disvaluing activities occur throughout the supply chain. The raw sugar is sent to a refinery, which further disvalues the product by refining it into white or brown sugar, incurring an extra disvaluing levy calculation of 8 percent that would be assessed on the refining company revenue. At the distribution and retail stages, there is no further disvaluation. The state and local sales taxes will not change and will be applied to the final sales price.

We have calculated the levy for raw sugar cane. Approximately 14 activities and 4 chemicals are used in creating raw sugar from the sugar cane plant; they result in a levy of 15 percent for raw sugar. The levy will apply to the raw sugar manufacturer revenue. Be aware that most people use their sugar refined and bleached into brown or white sugar, and the additional refining process would add another levy of 8 percent for the refining process. The 8 percent levy will apply to manufacturer revenue for refined white or brown sugar. The more these food products are processed, the more harmful compounds are used, and the more activities performed, the higher the levy percentage. High-fructose corn syrup is the same as sugar (actually, worse). It will have a similar levy calculation but a higher rate because of the level of activities and chemicals in the manufacturing process.

Unrefined raw sugar, or non-centrifugal sugar, is a product that has not been through any refining and still contains molasses with all its nutrients. There are only six disvaluing activities in processing unrefined NCS sugar, and no chemicals added. NCS sugar uses fewer than half of the raw sugar activity processes and no chemicals, resulting in an EDAL of 3 percent on the manufacturer's revenue.

As you can see from these raw and unrefined NCS sugar cane examples, using fewer activities and compounds to disvalue a product results in a much lower EDAL percentage. It is beyond comprehension why the sugar industry continues to refine its product to a level that increases its cost and strips the sugar cane of its nutrients and some of its sweetness.

If food company executives do not agree to reduce the harmful compounds in their processed foods voluntarily, then the only alternative is the tax route. They may try to slow legislation on the levy in Congress using their lobbyists, but we speculate that Congress may like the levy's approach to corporate revenue.

If lobbyists delay congressional legislation, another alternative is to have state legislatures enact the EDAL based on the PFTA list of compounds and activities. The PFTA can calculate the appropriate levy and recommend the calculations to each state legislature to make the levies uniform throughout the country. States influenced by food companies' lobbyists can continue to pay for Medicaid and other health programs from their general tax revenues. People can be made aware of the legislature's lack of action. The food companies' lobbyists in the U.S. Congress can target one governmental body; in the states, they will have to target 50 state legislatures and the governing bodies of Washington, DC, and Puerto Rico simultaneously. This approach is not the best situation, but in dealing with taxes, it is never pleasant.

§ § §

CHAPTER 13.

NATIONAL HEALTHCARE COSTS AND POTENTIAL SAVINGS

It is a fact that the food environment in the United States is affecting the health of all Americans of all ages. It is also a fact that metabolic syndrome diseases can be arrested and even reversed at a national level in a healthy living environment that includes healthy nutrition and exercise; the Cuban experience has proven it.

Healthcare Costs: Economic Implications for the Nation

As we have described in previous chapters, the chronic metabolic syndrome diseases have significant health and economic costs in the United States. Preventing and curing chronic diseases can reduce those costs significantly.

The following healthcare statistics should impress upon us the tremendous cost of metabolic syndrome to our country. We need to note the costs of the four leading chronic diseases, (1) cardiovascular disease, (2) cancer, (3) diabetes (type 2 diabetes), and (4) obesity. The total annual cost of just these four diseases adds up to over $1 trillion. There are other chronic diseases in the metabolic syndrome that are not included in that amount.

The debate in the 1960s and 1970s was about reducing our consumption of meat and saturated fat to 10 percent to prevent high cholesterol, heart disease, and strokes. By the end of the 20th century, we had accomplished that goal. Today, the number one killer of Americans is still heart disease, however. More than 868,000 Americans die of heart disease or strokes every year—that's one-third of all deaths in the United States. Heart diseases cost our healthcare system $214 billion per year and cause $138 billion in job productivity losses.[20]

The second most common killer in the United States is cancer. Almost 600,000 die from it every year, and more than 1.7 million people are diagnosed with cancer annually. Cancer care costs continue to rise and are expected to reach almost $174 billion by 2020. The job productivity losses are about 60 percent of the healthcare costs or $104 billion.[115]

The most prevalent metabolic syndrome disease is type 2 diabetes. More than 34.2 million Americans have it, and another 88 million adults in the United States have a condition called prediabetes, which puts them at significant risk for type 2 diabetes. In 2017, the total estimated cost of diagnosed diabetes was $327 billion in medical expenses and lost productivity.[21] This figure is growing at approximately 4 percent per year.

Obesity affects 19 percent of children and 42 percent of adults, and it puts people at risk for chronic diseases such as diabetes, heart disease, and cancer. Over a quarter of all Americans aged 17 to 24 years are too heavy to join the military. Obesity costs the U.S. healthcare system $147 billion a year and about $80 billion in lost productivity.[22]

Arthritis affects 54.4 million adults in the United States or approximately 1 in 4 adults. It is a leading cause of work disability in our country and one of the most common chronic conditions, as well as a common cause of chronic joint pain. Modern humans have evolved to have a specific ratio of omega-3 to omega-6 fatty acids. While this ratio varied slightly among populations, it is thought to have been about 1:1 throughout our human evolution. Excess omega-6 fatty acids in comparison to omega-3 fatty acids result in chronic inflammation leading to arthritis and other chronic diseases. Due to the Western diet, this ratio has changed significantly over the last century, and it may now be as high as 15:1 in the United States population. In 2013 the medical cost was $140 billion, and the cost of lost wages was $164 billion. It is estimated that those costs have increased at least 12 percent in the last 7 years.[23]

A 2017 survey of 11 developed countries' healthcare systems found the U.S. healthcare system to be the most expensive and worst-performing in terms of health access and equity. However, it is more advanced than the majority of developed countries. In a 2018 study, the United States ranked 29th in healthcare access to low-income groups. These surveys are not neutral and have built-in biases depending on the survey's group or organization.

Potential Healthcare Savings

Suppose we try to achieve what Cuba attained in 5 years. That would be a significant accomplishment for America. We can develop some estimates based on the statistics from Cuba and the cost of metabolic syndrome sicknesses in the United States. Let us begin by assuming the annual cost of a particular disease, in this case, cardiovascular disease. According to the U.S. costs quoted above, the yearly amount is $214 billion per year for healthcare and $138 billion in job productivity losses, for a total of $352 billion. In Cuba, cardiovascular disease incidence and mortality rates were reduced by 34.4 percent over 5 years, or 6.5 percent per year. If we calculate 6.5 percent of the $352 billion in U.S. annual costs, we will find that this country's potential reduction of costs can be $23 billion per year.

Diabetes in the United States in 2020 has an annual cost of approximately $367 billion. Suppose we multiply that number by the percentage of the yearly Cuban reduction in the prevalence and mortality rates of the disease, or 13.95 percent. In that case, we could potentially have savings in the United States of $51 billion per year.

The costs of healthcare and lost productivity due to cancer in the United States add up to $278 billion annually. The decrease in

Cuba's incidence and mortality rates of cancer was 2.4 percent, or a possible savings of $7 billion per year in the United States.

Obesity costs the United States $147 billion for healthcare and $80 billion in lost productivity and wages, for a total of $227 billion per year. The research reported an average weight loss in Cuba of about 12 pounds in 50 percent of the population. If the total number of overweight people in the United States costs the country $227 per year and could save 50 percent of those costs, the savings would amount to $114 billion annually.

By applying the statistics from the estimated Cuban reductions in illnesses to the United States healthcare and labor productivity costs, we can save, on the four diseases mentioned above, $195 billion per year. It would be a substantial reduction in our welfare costs, which have been increasing year after year. These estimates do not include some of the other chronic diseases of metabolic syndrome. We know the experts will say that we are making too many assumptions, but it is still a considerable amount even if we save only half of that amount, or approximately $100 billion a year. The potential savings will reduce the expenditures for Medicaid, the ACA, Medicare, and some private health insurance fees, helping alleviate healthcare costs.

We must act immediately to reduce healthcare expenses. The most ethical way to do so is to make our people healthier by decreasing our reliance on the Western diet of processed foods, as recommended in this book. Healthcare spending trends continue to rise. In 2019, healthcare spending in the United States grew by 4.6 percent to $3.8 trillion, or $11,582 per person. This pace of increase is consistent with that of 2018 (4.7 percent); see next section below. With the Covid-19 epidemic, healthcare expense growth rates will skyrocket in 2020 and 2021. According to some projections, growth will be in the double digits in 2020 and 2021. Our country cannot continue to spend so much money on healthcare and safeguard the profits of the processed food business. Assume our leaders lack the moral fortitude to act and instead hide behind the deceptive rhetoric of the processed food business. In that scenario, people need to take control of their health by avoiding processed meals altogether and consuming more natural foods.

Traditional Healthcare Benefits: Day of Reckoning?

One unavoidable truth that well-intentioned people may not want to hear is the economic reality of our healthcare system. Our country cannot afford to add another 30-plus million uninsured people to the healthcare rolls.[14] Our nation's population will grow by another 100 million people in the next 50 years, and the country cannot afford to add another 50 or 60 million sick people to the healthcare rolls.[116] It will bankrupt the system.

You may argue that increasing taxes can sustain the influx of additional people. We don't think politicians who want to be reelected will risk the significant tax increase required to keep the system solvent with all the extra people that will get sick. Healthcare costs have increased substantially in the United States.

- In 1960, healthcare costs were 5 percent of the GDP
- In 2018, they rose to $3.6 trillion, or 18 percent of the GDP; this was a 3.5 times increase in almost 48 years or $11,000 per person.[4] In 2019, it was **$11,582 per person per year.**
- By 2028, the current projection is an increase to $6.2 trillion, or 21 percent of the GDP, and $18,000 per person. This amount does not include the costs of Covid-19.[4]
- The Medicare Hospital Insurance Trust is projected to run out of money in 2026. Taxes will undoubtedly have to be increased because these projections have not considered the Covid-19 costs.[4, 19]
- By 2035, the Social Security funds for retirement and disability benefits will be gone. This program runs short of funds every year, and general taxes must be used to make the difference from the payroll tax shortfall. The Covid-19 costs are not included in the above numbers.[19, 117] They will significantly impact that projection, causing the day of reckoning to come sooner than projected, in 2025. Without a massive tax increase in payroll wages, Social Security as we know it will not be in place.

The year 2025 will be the year of reckoning for the American people. Four major healthcare factors will converge on that year:

1. There will be a continued increase in metabolic syndrome and the chronic diseases associated with it.
2. The early depletion of Social Security benefits will require massive payroll tax increases.
3. Only tax increases can replenish the Medicare hospital insurance depletions.
4. The expenses of Covid-19 will not have been recovered, and new virus variants will add additional costs well into 2022. The government will have to increase taxes to make up for the shortfall.

The national economy will not have recovered from the Covid-19 pandemic, especially the small business economy, which is the driving force of economic growth and employment. The massive fiscal expenditures in 2020 and 2021 will lead to inflation on the basic necessities diminishing the incomes for the low- and middle-income cohorts. People will begin to feel the effects of health-related social programs in 2023 and 2024, just before the presidential election, and politicians will seek someone to blame. They won't be able to blame their constituents for being sick, so they'll point the finger at the food companies for causing a chronic disease pandemic with their processed foods. They'll look at Asian countries where the population was healthy before the introduction of the Western diet. They will come to the same conclusion as we have: we need a new healthy approach to our food environment and a change in people's eating behavior.

Now that you know the background of this national health calamity, the obvious question is, what can we do? Throughout this book, we presented recommendations and strategies for handling this national emergency before it destroys our country. Now is the time for "we the people" to aid our country by changing our eating behavior, becoming healthier for our generation and the generations that follow.

§ § §

We have come to the end of the central theme of the book.

We tried to balance a concise presentation of the events leading to our health calamity with our recommendations for dealing with the crisis without including an overwhelming amount of in-depth detail. We hope we have accomplished that objective. You can read the appendices for more detailed information.

We want the people to be healthy. Future generations deserve it, and the country needs to start cultivating healthier nutritional trends now. We think this book's recommendations are vital for our country's future. So please spread the word among your family and friends and write a positive book review if you are so inclined.

The light of hope for our nation is bright if we can overcome the darkness of the health calamity.

§ § §

* * * * * * * * * * * * * * *

APPENDICES

APPENDIX A.

CUBA: A BRIEF HISTORY OF KEY EVENTS

A.1. Cuba: Accidental Health Crisis Briefing

The dissolution of the Soviet Union, the most significant global event of the second half of the 20th century, hit without warning. Its effect on Cuba was to initiate the worst economic and health crisis in the country's history. Cuba had been overly dependent on aid from the Soviet bloc, and when the aid ended abruptly, the Cuban nation was unprepared. The fact that the country survived is a testament to its people's resourcefulness and capacity for suffering and sacrifice. Cubans are highly innovative risk-takers and entrepreneurs.

Cubans are remarkable people who have struggled for independence and freedom since colonial times and continue to do so today. Cuba has a deluded ruling class that believes they are the only ones with the knowledge, wisdom, and understanding to control and rule society from the top down. Cuba is a centralized totalitarian regime that has destroyed people's human rights and victimized the population. Cubans would be one of the most successful Latin American countries if Cuba's ruling elite could stay out of the way and allow the people to apply their creativity freely.

The struggle in the 1990s was to survive with few food resources and few modes of transportation. The economic crisis created an extraordinary **accidental health** benefit. As a result, many Cubans lost weight, and the incidence and mortality rates of diabetes, heart disease, and cancer were significantly reduced. This health **breakthrough** was especially consequential because it included the entire nation's population.

Appendices A2, A3, and A4 will discuss Cuba's economic and health crisis of the 1990s. We provide historical background on Cuba and how the United States and Cuba have influenced each other over the centuries. Cubans refer to the 1990s as the "special period," the worst economic crisis in the island's history.[118] The situation occurred due to external political circumstances and the Cuban government's inability to adopt economic reforms that minimized the effects of the crisis on its people. Although Cuba is a totalitarian communist regime, our interest is not the political scene but, instead, the health of the Cuban people. This period saw a unique health scenario that has had no parallel in modern history, and its lessons for health in the United States form the premise of this book.

§ §

A.2. Cuba: Events Leading to the 1990s Crisis

The histories of Cuba[119] and the United States[120] are intertwined: One was a colony of the Kingdom of Spain and the other the colony of the United Kingdom of Britain, and both eventually became independent republics. To better understand why Cuba experienced a crisis in the 1990s, we provide a brief history covering the key events that led to that crisis.

1492:

Cuba was discovered by Christopher Columbus (Spanish: Cristóbal Colón) on October 28, 1492. The island became a critical possession of the Spanish Empire. Havana became the most important port in the Caribbean, and from it, Spanish ships sailed back to Spain carrying the treasures (mainly gold and silver) misappropriated from the South and Central American and Caribbean indigenous people. Spain became a global empire due to the riches in the Americas, especially central and south America.[119, 121]

1514:

In 1511, the Spanish crown decided to colonize the island of Cuba and sent Diego Velázquez de Cuèllar to subdue its local native population. After savagely massacring many unarmed Siboney and

Taino indigenous people in various battles, Velázquez enslaved the ones left to work the land and mines. In 1514 Cuba became an official colony of Spain. Velázquez was named its first governor, and by 1550 there were no native people left alive in Cuba. The Spaniards needed new slaves to work in the sugar cane fields, so they began to trade slaves from Africa, with the first ship arriving in Cuba in 1526.[122]

1762:

On August 13, 1762, after a 5-month siege, the British occupied and controlled Havana, the most strategic harbor in the Spanish West Indies. Havana was returned to Spain due to the first Treaty of Paris, signed in February 1763; in it, Spain ceded Florida to Great Britain in exchange for the city of Havana. At that time, the port of Havana was more strategically crucial to Spain than Florida was. Cuba was also a significant source of raw sugar cane for Spain in the 18th and 19th centuries.[121]

1902:

Cuba became an independent nation in 1902.[122, 123] Cuba's War of Independence, 1895 to 1898, was the last of three liberation wars that Cubans (Spanish and African descendants) fought against Spain. José Martí, the leader and symbol of Cuba's bid for independence from the Spanish Empire, was killed in the war's first battle on May 19, 1895.[124] In the final 3 months of the war, the United States got involved after the USS *Maine* exploded and sank in Havana harbor in 1898, and it defeated Spain in what is known as the Spanish-American War.[124, 125]

American forces were deployed in Cuba, Puerto Rico, and the Philippines. On December 18, 1898, the United States and Spain signed the second Treaty of Paris, giving Cuba its independence and ceding Puerto Rico and the Philippines to the United States. The United States did not grant freedom to Cuba immediately but waited until 1902, when democratic elections were held.[125]

1925:

Gerardo Machado was one of the Cuban War of Independence's youngest generals. In 1925, he was elected President. In an effort to modernize the country, the new president launched a series of successful projects. He was re-elected in fraudulent elections in 1929. His second term was violent and corrupt. The violence that surrounded him instilled fear in the Cuban people. His police brutally crushed all opposition. In 1933, the United States intervened and deposed Machado, establishing a provisional government. In the same year, an army sergeant, Fulgencio Batista, led a military coup in which the armed forces sergeants successfully overthrew the interim government. The sergeants form a five-man junta of four civilians and one military; Batista was the military member. Batista rose through the ranks of the Cuban military over the next few years to become the head of the Armed Forces.[122, 126]

1940:

This decade in Cuba sparked a chain of political events culminating in the Cuban revolution and the 1990s health crisis. We begin with Batista, who was a poor young African Cuban man of humble background. Both his parents were of mixed race, African, Spanish, Chinese, and one may have had indigenous blood. Batista joined the armed forces and was the leader of the sergeants' revolt of 1933. As the head of the Armed Forces in 1940, he ran for president and was popularly elected. Batista was a popular and strong leader. People thought of him as one of them. His initial popularity stemmed from his status as a mulatto symbol of Cuba's melting pot. Batista governed for his elected term, four years. Ramón Grau San Martin defeated him in the 1944 presidential elections. To this day, Batista is the only Cuban of African descent who has risen to the pinnacle of power in Cuba; no other African Cuban has reached such heights in the 60 years since the revolution began.[126]

1952:

In 1948, Carlos Prío Socarrás was elected President. His term in office was marked by corruption, and violence in the country, particularly between political parties. When the 1952 elections were marred by more violence, Batista saw an opportunity to seize power through a military coup. After successfully overthrowing Prío Socarrás, Batista installed himself as president. His leadership style, unfortunately, was not the same as when he was an elected president. He did not tolerate any criticism of his government and used the police to terrorize ordinary citizens. Unemployment became widespread throughout the country, with many university graduates unable to find work. Batista made a mistake by keeping intellectuals and the middle class out of government power. Despite romantic notions of a proletarian revolution, the revolution's leaders were middle-class, educated people who felt left out of government power. The time had come for a political shift.[126]

1953:

Fidel Castro had political ambitions and was becoming active in Cuban party politics in the 1952 elections. Who is Fidel Castro? Ángel Castro, Fidel's father, was an immigrant from Galicia, Spain, and a former soldier that fought for the Spanish Empire in Cuba. He went back to Spain after Cuba won its independence. He arrived back in Cuba in 1908, and by the time Castro was born, he had become a major sugar plantation landowner in Eastern Cuba. Fidel was educated mainly by private tutors and attended Colegio de Belen, a Jesuit Catholic private high school near Havana. He attended the University of Havana and majored in law.[121, 126, 127]

After Batista's illegal takeover of the presidency in 1952, Castro tried through legal means to remove Batista from power but failed. With no other option to participate in Cuban politics, Fidel Castro and his brother Raul attacked the Moncada Army Barracks (Cuartel Moncada) in Santiago de Cuba on July 26, 1953, accompanied by approximately 135 poorly trained Cubans. They aimed to take the second-largest city in Cuba and start a revolution to overthrow the Batista regime. The attack failed, and Fidel Castro and his brother were captured. Fidel Castro was tried and sentenced to 10 years in prison.[127] In prison, Castro immersed himself in Marxist-Leninist literature at the behest of his brother, Raul. He was released under an amnesty for political prisoners two years later and fled the country.

1956:

A revolutionary movement was born while Fidel Castro was in prison. He named the movement MR-26-7 in honor of the Moncada Army Barracks attack, which began the Cuban revolution.[127] After leaving Cuba, he went to Mexico and organized a group of Cubans to train as guerrillas fighters. They intended to land in the Eastern part of the island, in the same region as his father's sugar plantation. They planned to hike to the mountains and launch their revolutionary campaign. In December 1956, with a group of 82 Cubans, Fidel Castro landed on the Playa Las Coloradas (Coloradas Beach) near the town of Niquero to begin the revolutionary war in the Sierra Maestra the highest mountain range in Cuba.[126]

1959:

A second battlefront was opened in the Escambray mountains in the middle of the country in late 1958. Camilo Cienfuegos, a revolutionary commander, led the forces that took the city of Santa Clara near the mountains on December 31, 1958. Ernesto "Che" Guevara was a leader of a rebel column that supported Camilo Cienfuegos in his assault on the city. On January 1, 1959, a day after losing the city of Santa Clara, Cuban tyrant Batista left the country for fear of his life. The revolutionary forces of Fidel Castro declared Cuba's liberation from the Sierra Maestra mountain range. They arrived in Havana a few days later, after the Student Revolutionary Directorate had pacified the city.[127] Camilo Cienfuegos was named commander-in-chief of Cuba's armed forces shortly after the rebel army's victory in 1959. Raul Castro and Ernesto "Che" Guevara became Fidel Castro's trusted advisors because they shared Marxist beliefs. Both were staunch communists.

Ernesto "Che" Guevara was a loyal communist who was tasked with eliminating the opposition to the Castro regime. He presided over several Kangaroo trials (unfair show trials of political enemies, ignoring the law) and sentenced many dissidents to be shot. Guevara was equally zealous and ruthless in defending the revolution and had no compunctions about killing the dissidents. A few years later, bored with governing, he began organizing a mountain guerilla group in Bolivia to start a Communist revolution. Bolivian farmers did not support Guevara or his group; they were considered outsiders. The farmers assisted the Bolivian army in tracking the group.

According to army intelligence reports, Guevara asked the Castro brothers for help but was diplomatically told none would be forthcoming. Eventually, The Bolivian army killed Ernesto "Che" Guevara. Despite the romanticization of communist sympathizers today, Ernesto "Che" Guevara failed in his sole attempt to organize a communist revolution. He murdered many people in Cuba who spoke against Communism, as well as many Bolivians. If Guevara had been successful, he would have killed many more people in the cause of Communism. Ernesto "Che" Guevara followed in the footsteps of communist tyrants such as Joseph Stalin in Russia, Mao Zedong in China, Pol Pot of Cambodia's Khmer Rouge, and Kim Jong-un of North Korea. All of those men were or are communist tyrants who killed millions of their fellow countrymen in order to preserve power. Communist supporters use democracies' liberties to spread their utopian rhetoric, but the reality of communist governments must be scrutinized. Communist leaders have been the most heinous killers against their people in human history.

1960:

After overthrowing Fulgencio Batista, Fidel Castro began to show his communist leanings by confiscating private property. After Cuba seized American-owned Cuban oil refineries without compensation in October 1960, the United States placed an embargo on exports to Cuba except for food and medicine.[128] In Cuba, the embargo is called *el bloqueo* (the blockade). The embargo prevented American and foreign companies conducting business in the United States from trading with Cuba.

Fidel Castro responded with the confiscation and nationalization of the remaining American companies with no compensation. Simultaneously, the Cuban government confiscated all private property, including farmland, from the Cuban farmers who became salary workers in their former farms. Private property ceased to exist in Cuba. The embargo remains to this day and prevents trade between the two countries.

Opposition began to emerge among previous revolution sympathizers due to growing dissatisfaction with the communist principles that were being implemented. The regime labeled the dissidents as counter-revolutionaries. Castro established a network of neighborhood committees across Cuba in September 1960. The organizations, dubbed the "eyes and ears of the Revolution," exist to promote social welfare and report counter-revolutionary activities. The network was known as the "Committees for the Defense of the Revolution" (Comités de Defensa de la Revolución, or CDR). Fidel Castro called it a "collective system of revolutionary vigilance." It was established so that everybody knows who lives on every city block, what they do on every block, what relations they have had with counter-revolutionaries (dissidents), what activities they are involved in, and with whom they meet." The committees effectively gave the regime total control over the population.[126]

1961:

In April 1961, anti-Castro Cubans, supported by the United States, landed on the island at the Bay of Pigs.[129] The invasion, planned under Eisenhower but approved by Kennedy in his first few months as president, was allowed to fail when Kennedy withheld additional military support. After the failed invasion, Fidel Castro declared publicly that he and the island of Cuba were Marxist-

Leninist (i.e., communist) and aligned Cuba with the Soviet Union.[126]

Cuba's history is characterized by economic dependence on outside powers—first, Spain, then the United States, and now the Soviet Union. Fidel Castro had criticized previous Cuban governments for being servants *(lacayos)* of the United States, but he contradicted himself by becoming a "puppet" of the Soviet Union. Throughout history, Cuban leaders have never been astute in dealing with foreign superpower politics to serve the Cuban people. However, they have been clever when it comes to their own personal gain. Fidel Castro was no exception.

Cuba is a developing country, and before the revolution, the literacy rate was 77 percent, predominantly in the cities. The Castro regime launched an education campaign for the rural areas of the country. They dispatched "literacy brigades" of young teachers from cities to the countryside. The plan was twofold: first, to break down social barriers, the teachers, who mainly taught in cities, would realize the farmers and their families' living conditions. Second, to indoctrinate the illiterate population on the principles of Marxism-Leninism using the teaching books and pamphlets. According to UNESCO, the literacy rate for those over 15 years of age in Cuba was 99 percent in 2010. Economists at Oxford University's Our World In Data project calculated that during the same 50-year period (1960–2010), Latin America and the Caribbean's literacy rate increased from an average of 60% to 93% without the need for communists brigades.

The José Martí Pioneer Organization (Organización de Pioneros José Mart or OPJM) is a Cuban youth organization founded in 1961 to replace the banned Cuban Boy Scouts (Asociación de Scouts de Cuba). It is made up of primary and secondary students up to the ninth grade. José Martí, a Cuban writer and national hero, inspired the organization's name. The Young Pioneers are indoctrinated in communist ideology, taught to spy on their parents, and instructed to denounce them to their leaders. The organization's motto is: "Pioneers for communism: Let us be like Che!"[130]

As Cuba became more isolated from the United States, its dependency on Soviet aid and its communist satellites became more pervasive. Castro complained that Cuba could not be the master of its destiny with a United States historical chokehold on its economy. So he exchanged one superpower's control of Cuba's economy for another's.

1962:

In response to the failed Bay of Pigs invasion, Nikita Khrushchev, the Soviet leader, agreed to Fidel Castro's request to place nuclear missiles on Cuba to deter future aggression from the United States. In the summer of 1962, in Cuba, construction started on several atomic missile launch facilities.[129] After obtaining clear photographic evidence of the missile silos, the United States took action. Kennedy ordered a naval blockade on October 22nd to prevent further missiles from reaching Cuba. This action created a

United States confrontation with the Soviet Union, almost leading to a nuclear war.

After frantic negotiations between the United States and the Soviet Union, Kennedy and Khrushchev agreed that the Soviets would dismantle their missiles in Cuba and return them to the Soviet Union. The United States, in exchange, would make a declaration that it would not invade Cuba.[129] Historically, this event became known as the Cuban Missile Crisis, and it was as close as the world has been to a nuclear conflict. Nikita Khrushchev's act of nearly bringing the world to a nuclear confrontation cost him his job, and he was removed from power 2 years later.

1964-1974:

In later years Castro would tell an American reporter that he would not have hesitated to use the nuclear missiles against the United States. In other words, Castro was frustrated by his inability to influence superpower politics, in which he wanted to have a role.

American political leaders failed to understand the motivation of communist dictators. They looked at Fidel Castro through the prism of American politics and policies. They thought that material rewards offered by the United States to countries aligned within its sphere of influence were superior to what the Soviet Union could offer. American politicians surmised that the Cuban people would not stand for a communist dictatorship. They failed to realize that the most efficient component of a communist government is population indoctrination and control by preventing any regime criticism or dissent.

Fidel Castro was not a typical Latin American dictator who would bend to the will of the U.S. government or corporations. He was an ardent communist who challenged the United States on many political fronts in Latin America and Africa. In most cases, he was triumphant, to the detriment of U.S. international prestige. The U.S. political elite failed to grasp Fidel Castro's essence, absolute power, and cruelty in wielding power.

The Soviet Union offered that absolute power to Fidel Castro and supported his foray into Latin American and African politics. To this day, elite American politicians still do not grasp Latin American issues. In Venezuela, Cuban intelligence agents are keeping an inept president in power, which has brought the entire country down. Since Hugo Chávez and Nicolás Maduro took control, 6 million Venezuelans have sought refuge in neighboring countries like Colombia, Panama, and the United States.[131] The United States and its intelligence agencies seem to be on the sidelines, hoping for the government to crumble.

1980:

The years 1963 through early 1989 were relatively stable for Cuba in economic terms because the country was being heavily supported by Soviet aid. The exception was 1980, when an inflationary global energy crisis hit Cuba, creating a minor economic downturn. In the early 1980s, food became scarce, and riots occurred in some of the major cities. Groups of Cubans overran the gates of various Latin American embassies in Havana, seeking political refuge. These actions reached a peak when 10,000 Cubans sought refuge on the Peruvian embassy's grounds.

The Cuban government was confronted with an untenable political situation and needed to regain control of the cities. In a bold move, Castro announced that anyone who wanted to leave Cuba could do so. An understanding was reached with Cuban exiles in Miami that they could come by boat to the port of Mariel in northwestern Cuba and pick up their family and friends who wanted to leave the country.

The Mariel Boatlift lasted for 6 months, from April to October 1980. By the time Castro closed the doors again, 125,000 Cubans had left the island. The political pressure on the Cuban government was eased, and Fidel Castro discovered a new political tool that he could use whenever discontent erupted in the Cuban population. He would use it again when his regime was threatened.[132]

People with no hope of changing their situation are desperate people capable of taking violent action. If you give those same people some hope of changing their untenable conditions, the problem can be controlled. Fidel Castro allowed people to flee to stabilize the political situation in Cuba. This tactic worked for the next few years.

1989:

The economic situation changed again with the Union of Soviet Socialist Republics (USSR) breakup, which began in late

1989. The demise of the USSR started with the Polish constitution change in December of 1989 and the holding of subsequent free elections in 1990, establishing the Republic of Poland. This led to growing unrest in other Soviet Republics and culminated in the complete dissolution of the USSR in 1991.[15] The Eastern European republics stopped trading with Cuba, and the Soviet Union stopped sending any aid to Cuba.

As the liberated formerly communist republics began to adopt free-market reforms requiring payments in international currencies, Cuba's economic situation became a crisis.[133] This crisis was called the *special period* (*período especial*) and was a time of financial turmoil and widespread shortages in Cuba, most notably of food. Their reliance on an outside power once again haunted the Cuban people.

The early 1990s:

The economic crisis in the early 1990s led to significant riots in Cuba and threatened Cuba's political stability once again. In response, Fidel Castro announced that anyone who wished to leave the island could do so. A significant exodus of close to 40,000 Cubans sailed to the United States via makeshift rafts (*balseros*) over 5 weeks. Many thousands drowned on the homemade rafts in the swift gulf currents of the Florida Straits between Cuba and Florida.[134]

Although it was in many ways a tragic time for the Cuban people, the 1990s also turned out to be a unique milestone from a health perspective. The scarcity of food and fuel created a health crisis for the island of 11 million people, but the crisis had positive repercussions for their health. It may today provide us with some lessons for easing the current U.S. health calamity.

The year is **2021**, and Cuba's economy is once again in rapid collapse. There is again a lack of food. Cubans throughout the island are taking to the streets to protest a lack of liberty and 60 years of oppression. Protests are ruthlessly suppressed, but Marxist apologists have a dilemma. Protesters are comprised of young people, artists, poets, and writers. Young African Cubans sing for liberation. They have a slogan and a song that has become the anthem of the new revolutionaries, "Patria y Vida," which translates as "homeland and life." If Cuba is an equality paradise, why are young African Cubans and notably African Cubans artists, poets, and writers, at the vanguard of the protests and clamoring for freedom?

§ §

A.3. Cuba: Healthcare System: Doing More with Less

Cuba is the largest island in the Caribbean Sea, with scarce natural resources. The revolutionary government promised healthcare for all citizens but realized that it did not have the resources to treat every Cuban.[127, 135] A different approach to healthcare was needed to fulfill the constitution's mandate. The answer was to prevent citizens from getting sick. The first step was periodic medical check-ups for the general population. The government had to establish community clinics (consultorios), each with a family doctor, to achieve that goal.[135] The family doctor began compiling a medical history for each patient and updating it regularly (usually once a year). The government was now in the business of keeping people healthy.[136]

In most cases, doctors went out into the community to see patients, take their vital signs, and discuss their health concerns. Extensive questionnaires regarding occupations, family, housing situations, and community living were also included in those medical checkups. Over time, this proactive approach to medicine has become more efficient.[137] The program provided the communist regime additional control of the people by identifying each individual's illness and healthcare needs, financial situation, living conditions, and family allegiance. The government now controlled all aspects of economic, health, and social life.

The healthcare strategy revolves around a community clinic system that provides primary care from a local physician. The method differs from the more expensive illness treatment strategy used in the United States. Although the United States healthcare system is more advanced than Cuba's, it is a fragmented treatment fee system where patients are shuttled between medical specialists, laboratories, and hospitals. As a result, it is both more costly and inefficient than Cuba's healthcare system.[137] A note of caution: Almost any medical system for 11 million people will be significantly easier to manage than one for 330 million people.

The economic situation in Cuba has always been one of scarcity and hardship. For example, Cuba has had food rationing since the beginning of the revolution over 60 years ago. Family doctors in the community clinics manage to provide their services without access to the latest diagnostic technology.[138] It takes weeks for necessary medical supplies to arrive at the clinics and hospitals.[135]

Healthcare is not the same for all Cubans. One healthcare system for the general population and another for the Cuban elites (party members, military leaders, and official celebrities) have access to more advanced facilities and equipment. There is the so-called *medical tourism* for foreigners willing to pay in dollars or euros. The dual healthcare system reminds us of a quote from a book we read in our youth, a satire of the Soviet Union and its Marxist/Leninist political doctrine. In *Animal Farm* by George Orwell, published in 1945, the pigs who control the farm make the proclamation that "All animals are equal, but some animals are more equal than others."[139] The quote describes the reality of Cuba today and also other communist countries.

Statistics prove that Cuba's healthcare approach is working. Although Cuba is a developing country with scarce natural resources, the life expectancy of its citizens is about the same as in the United States: 78 years for men and 81 years for women.[135] However, this will soon change because life expectancy declined for the first time in U.S. history due to increased metabolic syndrome diseases.[6, 80] Cuba's infant mortality rate per thousand births of 4.2 is also comparable to that of more developed countries. However, Cuba is not immune to modern chronic diseases, and Cubans did not learn the lessons from the 1990s health crisis.

Although an accidental health benefit from the 1990s health crisis significantly reduced metabolic syndrome diseases by 2010, Cuba's type 2 diabetes, cardiovascular diseases, and cancer rates were at the pre-1990s levels.[3] Even with a preventive approach, healthcare workers could not stop metabolic syndrome diseases after 2010. The reason is that the Cuban diet is no longer healthy. Food continues to be scarce; people eat whatever is available, and unfortunately, what has become available is processed foods and sugary beverages. Cuba's recent experience provides more evidence of why the Western diet is detrimental to a nation's health. Preventive medicine in Cuba helps to identify metabolic syndrome once it is discovered but not to prevent it. Preventing the syndrome requires a healthy natural food environment, which was available in the 1990s during the food shortage but is no longer present. That is why metabolic syndrome diseases are back to pre-1990s levels.[3] The Cuban model does not prevent metabolic syndrome. However, the model appears to be effective once symptoms are identified and managed. In the United States, when the syndrome is diagnosed, it is treated and managed with medicines.

The preventive healthcare approach to medicine that works in Cuba has not been adopted by any other developing country. The healthcare model of today's Cuba works because of the country's totalitarian political regime. Its healthcare system emerged from the same efforts used to educate the people to eliminate illiteracy. Access to healthcare became another tool used to control and indoctrinate the people in communist ideology.

The preventive healthcare approach can work but becomes too expensive to apply with modern medical technology. Cuban doctors in community clinics do not apply all the modern techniques of doing a comprehensive blood test and other radiological and sonographic procedures that doctors in Western countries utilize. Cuban doctors rely on the patient's vital signs and their intuition and experience to make a diagnosis. Cuba provides healthcare with older medical technology and still spends nearly 7 to 8 percent of its gross domestic product on healthcare, a significant portion for a developing country.[135] It is not clear why the expenditure is so large. Perhaps it is because of the many doctors who graduate from Cuban universities and the number of doctors per capita.

As an island with almost no natural resources to export, Cuba has found a new export: medical doctors. Thousands of physicians graduate from Cuban universities each year, but most are sent to work in other nations. This scenario causes problems in the domestic healthcare system because the community clinic doctors that remain in Cuba are overworked. The government spends about $300 to $400 per person on healthcare each year, while doctors are paid less than $100 per month.[135]

Doctors who travel abroad are paid more, but the Cuban government takes a large portion of the foreign currency they earn (estimated to be between $8 and $10 billion annually).[140] Doctors and engineers in Cuba work as taxi drivers or waiters in tourist hotels because they earn more money from foreign tourists than government-employed doctors and engineers. Government funds are used to train professionals to work as low-skilled laborers, creating an upside-down economy.

Cuban doctors have provided medical services in Africa, South America, and Portugal, among other places. During the COVID-19 epidemic, they also offered medical assistance to Italy, Brazil, and China. Following the demise of the Soviet Union in 1991, international medical engagement increased. Thousands of Cuban healthcare professionals worked in Venezuela under Hugo Chávez in exchange for oil, and they continue to do so under the current government of Nicolás Maduro.[131]

In the 1990s in Venezuela, Cuba initiated a significant program to restore people's eyesight. In 2004, this medical program was extended to 14 other Latin American countries where people suffer from cataracts and other eye diseases.[141] In Uruguay, the Graduate School of the Faculty of Medicine has recently criticized Cuban doctors and made it known that they have failed to pass their ophthalmology test. The Cuban doctors have only specific ophthalmology expertise (like a technician) but lack the general knowledge of the specialization.[142] The government of Bolivia has complained that of the 702 Cuban doctors deployed in the country, only 205 have medical degrees; the rest are technicians.[142]

§ §

A.4. Cuba: Accidental Health Results and a Planned Economy

The 1990s were a time of economic turmoil and severe shortages in Cuba. Food shortage created a public health crisis affecting 11 million people across the country. Physicians who returned to Cuba after overseas medical missions between 1990 and 1992 found a very different country from what they had left a few years previously.[140] To understand how the economic crisis arose, we need some perspective on its causes. We'll start with the external (foreign) components.

The USSR's demise was precipitated by the secession of Eastern European communist countries from the USSR, which resulted in a change in Cuba's economic situation. Former Soviet states began the process of transitioning to free-market economies. They demanded that their trade contacts with Cuba be conducted using standard commercial practices rather than a barter system.[133] Therefore, Cuba's economic support from those communist countries disappeared almost overnight, along with the Soviet Union's aid.

Cuba's 5-year Economic Plans (Planned economy)

Even though the Soviet's help to former satellite countries ceased as well, the Soviet republics did not face the same difficulties as Cuba. Instead of the planned economy previously used in their countries, they switched to a free-market economy. Cuba was affected by external economic causes; domestic difficulties also played a role in the abrupt economic decline. The Castro regime's refusal to implement political and economic reforms exacerbated the financial situation. The crisis worsened the inefficiencies that came with a centrally planned economy and hastened the economic woes.

In a speech to the National Assembly, Fidel Castro declared the situation as “a special period in a time of peace” and said that the Cuban people would have to “tough it out” as if it were a time of war. In other words, the Cuban people would have to suffer further and survive the scarcity of food and fuel.

Because fuel oil was scarce in Cuba during the 1990s, buses, vehicles, and trucks vanished from the streets and highways. Cubans had to walk to work, rely on a few accessible horse-drawn carts, or ride one of the government's one million bicycles imported from China. Because there was no fuel oil for their farm equipment, farmers had to resort to manual farming methods. Farm production plummeted, and goods couldn't be transported to cities.

Permaculturists from other countries who had arrived in Cuba at the time taught their techniques to locals, who quickly applied them in fields, raised beds, and rooftop gardens around the country. Permaculture is an approach to land management and philosophy that adopts arrangements observed in flourishing natural ecosystems. Organic agriculture was implemented after the Cuban government enforced it due to a lack of funds to buy chemical fertilizers.[143] The government also supplied vegetable seeds for planting in urban gardens. Farmers in both the city and the country were required to deliver their produce to government agencies. Still, they were allowed to keep a portion for themselves and sell the remainder to the broader public, thereby indirectly acknowledging the black market.

For the first time since private farms were confiscated in 1960, the government has no choice but to approve land leases for small private farms to feed the populace. New land was offered near private farms to encourage families to build homes near their farms, help with food production, and sell their gathered goods and animal meats at local farmers' markets. Although starvation was avoided, persistent hunger became a daily occurrence, never observed before the Cuban Revolution.[3]

Farmland leasing and privatization have been implemented successfully in China and Vietnam. Private farmers are thriving because they can sell their goods at market prices. Vietnam can now feed the entire country with their farms' production. The Cuban government's dogmatic communists will not accept market prices and have fixed the price for every farm commodity grown by the private farmers. Many farmers are losing money, so they just farmed enough to keep the farm running and limit their losses. It illustrates the communist regime's inflexibility in Cuba, where doctrine takes precedence over people's well-being.

The Cuban government, like communist governments around the world, has the same blind spots. The leaders continue to believe that they are more intelligent than the general public and that, as a result, they are the only ones who can guide the country in a way that benefits the people. They reduced everyone to the lowest common denominator: poverty to promote equality among the people. That kind of "equality" in Cuba can also be seen in North Korea and Venezuela. Individuality, inventiveness, and entrepreneurship are all suppressed, and only one political philosophy and one planned economy are permitted. The Orwellian Big Brother (from George Orwell's novel *Nineteen Eighty-Four*) knows best in such a setting.

China saw the most drastic transition from a socialist centrally planned economy to a free-market economy. Vietnam has followed China by opening its economy to allow privatization. When the People's Republic of China took power in 1949, it ruled according to strong Marxist/Leninist principles. Mao Zedong established the government-run planned economy as a feature of socialist economies. After undertaking several government endeavors to industrialize China, including the "Great Leap Forward," which resulted in the country's worst famine in history, it was evident that Mao's communist approach to industrialized the country had failed.

Deng Xiaoping, a visionary and pragmatic leader of the Communist Party ostracized by Mao Zedong, realized that central planning did not work.[144] After Mao's death, he initiated reforms that rewarded self-enterprise and propelled the Chinese people from abysmal poverty to enormous wealth in less than 40 years, lifting

600 million people out of poverty at the same time.[145] That happened under a free-market economy, not a socialist planned economy.

Deng said, "Being poor is not socialism," and the Chinese people embraced this view. He is revered as the architect of modern China. He had read Adam Smith's *"The Theory of Moral Sentiments"* and *"The Wealth of Nations"* and applied Smith's free-market principles in China.[146]

The city of Shenzhen, established in 1980, grew from a fishing settlement of 80,000 people to a city of 12 million people in 2015 and is called the East's Silicon Valley. It was founded under Deng Xiaoping's policies as a free-market city. Today, China's success in switching from a centrally planned to a free-market economy has pushed China to become the world's second-largest economy after the United States.[145]

Why do we mention China? Although Cuba's leaders are admirers of the Chinese Communist Party, they did not learn the economic lessons of Deng Xiaoping and continued to adhere to old socialistic central-planning principles that exacerbated Cuba's financial crisis. The Cuban socialists were and are extreme Marxist/Leninist linear thinkers who rely on a discredited communist doctrine and bad economic practices. Making changes in their economy contradicts their socialistic logic. Consequently, Cuba continues to endure the worst financial and health crisis in its history. In 2021, riots and protests in the cities have again demanded more food and political freedom. Cuba's revolutionary slogan is "Patria o Muerte" (homeland or death), the protesters' slogan is "Patria y Vida" (homeland and life). Young African Cubans have a song named "Patria y Vida" that has become a freedom anthem for the young Cuban people. After 60 years of communism, their conditions have not improved, and they are asking how much longer they will have to wait to reap the benefits of the communist revolution. They have surrendered their freedom and endure a subsistence life of sacrifice while the rest of the world passes them by, leaving them with unfulfilled longing.

Mismanagement of Foreign Financial Aid

In the first 30 years after the revolution, Cuban leaders spent most of the financial aid from Russian and international banks on promoting revolutions in Africa and Latin America. They did not use it to create the industries and infrastructure that would have raised Cubans' living standards. As a result, Cuba's primary economic structure changed very little between 1959 and the 1990s. Tobacco products such as cigars and cigarettes were among Cuba's leading exports but were manufactured using a preindustrial process. The manufacture of raw sugar cane continued to decline over that period owing to a lack of modern manufacturing equipment and techniques.

The Cuban economy remained inefficient and produced only a few highly subsidized commodities by the Soviet bloc countries. The lack of investment in the economy is the reason the country is in a dire economic situation today. In 2016, Cuba defaulted on its foreign debt and requested a renegotiation of the loans. Russia forgave a portion of its loans, $32 billion, and the Europeans forgave $11 billion, and new terms were negotiated.[147] In 2019, Cuba defaulted on the renegotiated loans but promised to pay its debts in the next few years. As of this writing, the debts have not been paid.

The Cuban government suppresses all entrepreneurial endeavors, essentially removing the population segment that generates new ideas. For example, restaurant permits are in high demand, yet the government has ceased providing them without reason or rationale. Because the government has not invested in new equipment, raw sugar production has decreased. Without a significant investment in new equipment, unrefined sugar (non-centrifugal cane sugar) can be produced utilizing some of the old sugar mills' equipment; all they need are the available cold-presses.

Small entrepreneurs in Colombia, Brazil, India, and Indonesia produce unrefined sugar (NCS) because they do not need a centrifuge or expensive equipment. These entrepreneurs are creating new markets in health-conscious countries. Cuba's front-end sugar mill equipment continues to rust away because the government cannot adapt to a free-market system as China and Vietnam have done. Small entrepreneurs adapt and change to help the economy in other countries, but in Cuba, pointless 5-year economic plans do not work and never come to fruition.

The 1990s Health Crisis and Its Implications

Now that we've provided some historical context, you can see how the Cuban crisis of the 1990s presented a unique opportunity for medical researchers. It was a situation brought about by ineffective government policies rather than by war or famine. In 2007, the *American Journal of Epidemiology* released the sole scholarly study we could find on health issues in Cuba during this timeframe. The researchers came from Baltimore's Johns Hopkins School of Public Health, Chicago's Loyola University, and Cienfuegos, Cuba's University Hospital.[2]

Their updated research appeared in the *British Medical Journal* in April 2013. Like every research document, the title is a mouthful: "Population-wide Weight Loss and Regain in Relation to Diabetes Burden and Cardiovascular Mortality in Cuba 1980-2010: Repeated Cross-Sectional Surveys and Ecological Comparison of Secular Trends."[3]

The research objective was to evaluate the associations between population-wide weight loss and gain and the prevalence, incidence, and mortality rates of diabetes, cardiovascular disease, and cancer in Cuba over a 30-year interval. One of the key findings was that between 1990 and 1995, Cubans, in general, consumed fewer calories than they expended each day. They were very physically active due to the effort required to bicycle, walk to work, or go to a grocery store.[3] According to the research measurements, the calorie expenditure versus consumption led to an average weight loss of 12 pounds (5.5 kg) in most adults during the first half of the 1990s.[3]

Twelve pounds or more is a significant number in a national population. But most significantly and essential, the people's health improved, and the death rates of chronic diseases plunged. The death rate from diabetes was cut in half, and deaths from heart disease were cut by one-third. There was a 2.4 percent decline in cancer mortality rates.[2]

The accidental health crisis in Cuba indicates that weight loss in the general population and an appropriate diet can positively impact health relatively quickly. During that period, the weight loss was attributed to fewer calories and the increased physical activity.[3] However, the researchers did not consider three key variables that could explain the health results more comprehensively, although they mentioned them indirectly. They are (1) a natural food environment, (2) time-restricted feeding, (3) and intermittent fasting. We discussed those factors in Chapter 02.

The researchers seemed to focus basically on calories (energy). The biochemistry of calories is too complex to explain the weight loss achieved and the positive health results.[24] We know from randomized trials that expending more calories than we consume does not necessarily lead to long-term weight loss because our metabolism adapts to the lower caloric intake.[32, 148] Focusing on food choices as a variable would have provided a more reliable measurement of the reversal of metabolic syndrome diseases.

Explaining the weight loss based on the type of food consumed would have been better than the calories-in, calories-out explanation. A lack of petroleum during the 1990s affected travel, commuting, electrical power generation, food processing, and beverage production. Therefore, processed foods, vegetable oils, sugary beverages, and their transportation for distribution were not available.

The researchers hinted at diet when they referenced the farmers' ability to sell directly to the public. The growth of urban farming in the cities and suburbs increased the available nutrients from green vegetables. The lack of food choices led to a natural food environment of primarily green vegetables, although chicken, pork, and locally caught wild fish were available in the black market. The black market was pervasive and, in effect, a second economy. The researchers also hinted at inadvertent intermittent fasting and time-restricted feeding. They noted that although starvation was avoided, persistent hunger was a fact of life not seen since before the revolution.[3] In our interviews of Cubans that lived through that period, they stated that there were days with no food, and when food was available, they would eat once or twice a day to conserve food.

The Cuban government requires citizens to use a grocery food booklet (*libreta de abastecimiento*) to buy food in government grocery stores. The government establishes the amount and frequency of food each person can buy.[149] The food distribution system has been in place for almost 60 years. The scarcity of food in the 1990s did not result in periods of starvation, but there were many days on which people ate only one meal a day and, at times, did not have anything to eat for a few days. Milk was scarce and reserved only for children.

We know that our metabolism can adjust to an intake of fewer calories, preventing a significant weight loss from a low-calorie diet.[100] The calories and nutrients Cubans ate mainly were from vegetables and meats. Dr. Jason Fung's research on obesity and diabetes can help explain the Cuban's reductions in weight and lowered death rates due to type 2 diabetes and associated hypertension.[24, 37]

In summary:

- Over 5 years, many Cubans lost an average of 12 pounds or more, and most Cubans were normal-weight people.
- The weight loss was attributed to food scarcity, a low caloric intake, and high caloric expenditure, but this was not the whole story. We know from randomized trials that expending more calories than we consume does not lead to long-term weight loss because our metabolism adapts to the lower caloric intake.
- Processed foods, vegetable oils, sugars, and sugary beverages were unavailable during those 5 years due to a lack of electricity for running factories and fuel oil for transport.

- During those 5 years, the Cuban diet included natural foods such as green vegetables and (occasionally) chicken, pork, and locally caught wild fish available on an active and pervasive black market. Thus, by accident, a natural food environment was generated. Milk was reserved for children.
- In general, people ate one or two meals a day on most days, and some days, they ate no meals at all.
- Diabetes mortality rates were cut in half during that period, and there was also a reduction in the incidence of type 2 diabetes.
- Cardiovascular mortality rates were reduced by one-third.
- Cancer mortality rates were reduced by 2.4 percent.

Cuba did not learn the lessons that the 1990s health benefits offered. It was a painful period for Cubans that they would rather forget. The government did not understand the health benefits to their nation. It did not educate the population on the advantages of a natural food environment. The proof is in the updated research comments toward the end of their 2013 article. The data showed that towards the end of the 1990s, as fuel and food became more available, the population started to gain weight. The incidence of diabetes increased, along with the mortality rate.[3] The production of processed foods with oils and sugar, and sugary beverages also increased during this period. By the beginning of 2002, mortality rates had returned to earlier higher levels. A particularly dramatic shift in diabetes mortality rates was observed: From 2002 to 2010, the annual increase in type 2 diabetes matched the rate before the health crisis. Rates of coronary heart disease and strokes were also similar to those before the crisis.[3]

It is an interesting paradox that even though Cubans tend not to be obese, rates of metabolic syndrome are once again high in the population. This observation supports Dr. Lustig's research findings that obesity does not cause metabolic syndrome but is just a marker of it.[29] Other substances cause metabolic syndrome diseases in the Cuban population, such as sugary drinks that cause fatty liver leading to insulin resistance, type 2 diabetes. Unhealthy processed foods are also the cause of other chronic diseases such as cardiovascular diseases. Food is still somewhat scarce in Cuba, and the population eats whatever foods are available.

§ §

Appendix B.

A Briefing on Human-Made Industrialized Food [7]

B.1. Industrialized Ultraprocessed Convenience Foods

Let's look at how the story of human-made processed food originated and progressed. Since the advent of the modern Industrial Revolution, we have had an abundance of food unprecedented in human history. In the 1800s, the food industry began introducing new food-processing methods, particularly the refining of grains and sugar, which impacted the Western diet. "Refined grain flour" is a remarkable early example of processed food. Wheat grains have an *endosperm* or starchy part; the *germ* contains protein, fat, and vitamins; and the *bran* contains fiber. During the refining process, the germ and bran are removed. The refined flour is made from the endosperm (starch) and is usually bleached to make it more appealing to consumers. That product is

7 Note: Some sentences may be repeated from previous chapters to provide continuity of content.

known as "white flour," which is a harmful factory-made food that spikes your blood sugar levels.

White bread, cake, doughnuts, and cereals are all made with white flour and partially hydrogenated (trans fat) vegetable oils. What reason, you may ask, did the food-processing industry have for removing the germ and bran? The answer is a longer shelf-life and retaining freshness during transportation. Grain has a shorter shelf-life if the nutrients and fiber are retained. The shelf-life is measured in years after the germ and bran have been removed. The first factory-processed fast food and the first chronic ailments had come with refined white flour.[8] How? Refined flour has little nutritional value, but it speeds up glucose metabolism in our bodies, resulting in fat excess and obesity, and spiking glucose levels.

In early 1921, the food industry began producing white bread in factories. White bread made with refined white flour was a significant factor in illnesses. White bread was the mainstay of poor children's diets due to its low cost. Many children developed rickets disease caused by a lack of vitamin D. According to scientists, the germ, which carried the vitamins, was removed from the grains during the flour refinement process. The manufacturer's approach was to reinsert synthetic vitamin D into white flour, the so-called enriched or fortified bread. Milk was also fortified with synthetic vitamin D.

The white bread episode was one of the first documented cases of harmful factory-processed food being produced. The fortified bread was hailed as a breakthrough in food preparation by the press. No one questioned why the vitamins were eliminated throughout the refining process in the first place. The public's response was to buy more white bread and believe the marketing claims of an industry's success. The company continues to make white bread fortified with vitamin D and other synthetic nutrients to this day. This action would be a watershed moment for processed food industries to address negative nutritional health issues in the future.

Western countries, particularly the United States, gradually improved factory food processing throughout the first half of the twentieth century. Proctor & Gamble introduced cottonseed oil (Crisco) in 1911 as a healthier alternative to lard or butter. Crisco shortening is hydrogenated trans fat, which is harmful and causes cardiovascular disease and strokes. Trans fat was eventually banned by the FDA in 2015, more than 100 years later and 50 years after the dangers of trans fats were discovered. Because seed oil does not sound particularly appetizing, the business refers to it as "vegetable oil." When heated beyond the smoke point, vegetable oils have been shown to generate carcinogens harmful to our health. The high omega-6 fat content contributes to cardiovascular illnesses, erectile dysfunction (ED), type 2 diabetes, and inflammation in our bodies.

As a result, the industry is considering changing the label to "plant oils." This name is more fitting in some respects, as the oils are produced in enormous chemical factories similar to oil refineries. We are, of course, being facetious.

The era of food processing industrialization has arrived. The ultraprocessed food industry did not become a major component of the food establishment until World War II. The food sector conducted most of its research on processed foods under the supervision of the US Army to produce the K-rations needed to sustain soldiers on the battlefield. Dr. Ancel Keys was a key figure in the invention of the K-rations. In the 1960s and 1970s, he will be remembered as a leading proponent of decreasing saturated fat to lower cholesterol and heart disease, giving birth to the low-fat, high-carb diet with devastating results.[5]

Following WWII, ultraprocessed foods began to emerge on grocery store shelves in greater numbers. Ultraprocessed foods were promoted as convenient and nutritious for a healthy nation. However, what exactly is ultraprocessed food? Carlos Monteiro, a Brazilian nutrition researcher, and his colleagues at the University of Sao Paulo were the first to conceive and develop the concept.[108] From their work emerged the NOVA classification of food and its four categories:

1. **Unprocessed or minimally processed foods** (think raw vegetables and dry beans or legumes, raw nuts, fresh-cut pasture-raised meat, fresh-caught wild fish, and frozen vegetables without added ingredients)
2. **Processed culinary ingredients** (think butter, lard, tallow, coconut fat, unrefined sugar or noncentrifugal cane sugar, and coarse or sea salt)

3. **Processed foods** (think canned vegetables and fruits, canned fish and meat, cheese, bread, bagels, beer, and wine, and salted or sugared nuts)
4. **Ultraprocessed foods and drinks (UPFDs)** (think chicken nuggets, hamburger sandwiches, twinkies, margarine, cakes, cookies, refined sugar, refined flour, pastries, candies, sugary beverages, fruit juices, breakfast cereals, hot dogs, pizza, sausages, instant soups, salad dressings, and sweets)[108]

Some of us remember the sugary beverage industry's attempt to confound us with a marketing campaign that stated that all calories are the same. Coca-Cola's advertising campaign of 2013, "Coming Together," was the culmination of such efforts. According to the campaign, a calorie is a calorie (all calories are the same), whether from Coca-Cola or broccoli.

When faced with the negative consequences of their products, food processors recalled the white bread lesson from the past. They unleashed their marketing machine to reply with a gimmick that muddled the public's understanding of the situation. The stratagem in the most recent of these campaigns is "freedom of choice.".[150] Freedom for the food companies to experiment with our health, not for the people assaulted with deceptive advertising propaganda across all communication mediums.

§ §

B.2. Industrialized Refined Sugar

Cuba was a major producer of raw sugar cane before the revolution, which many people are unaware of this fact. Currently, Brazil is the major producer of raw sugar. Some of the compounds that are lost in refined sugar are found in raw sugar cane. Cuba exports natural raw sugar, which is refined into light brown or white sugar in Europe and other countries, and stripped of any remaining nutrients. Although Cuba is no longer a major exporter of raw sugar cane, the crop remains an essential part of the Cuban economy.

Cuba is also a member of the International Sugar Organization (ISO).[151] The Cuban revolutionary government shut off the supply of raw sugar cane to the United States because of the 1961 Bay of Pigs incident. To keep refined sugar prices from rising, the United States sought a new sugar supplier. High-fructose corn syrup (HFCS), a sweetener like refined sugar (in fact, it's worse because it's 45 percent glucose and 55 percent fructose) but about half the price, was the substitute. This substitute benefits the United States economically, but it has been worst for the American people because it has been added to all kinds of processed food due to its lower price.

The production of raw sugar cane in Cuba fell during the 1990s crisis. To earn foreign currency, whatever was produced was exported, which meant that Cuban sugar consumption plummeted during this period. Sugary beverage bottlers could not make their products due to a scarcity of energy and transportation of fuel oil. Another critical health determinant in the fall of type 2 diabetes in Cuba was less consumption of refined sugar, which resulted in a 50 percent reduction in mortality. Insulin resistance, which leads to metabolic syndrome and type 2 diabetes, is exacerbated by refined sugar consumption.[1, 46]

Sugar cane has the same unfavorable consequences as refined wheat (white) flour. The wheat plant is a light-brown grain packed with minerals and fibers that are good for the human body in its natural state. However, the grain is stripped of its nutrients and fiber during the refining process to make white flour. Wheat flour that has been refined into white flour is unhealthy and spike blood sugar leading to insulin resistance.

Sugar cane refining is comparable to wheat flour. Sugar cane is a perennial grass that grows between 6 and 19 feet tall. It is the world's most abundant crop in volume, accounting for 79 percent of all refined sugar. Sucrose accumulates in the sugar cane plant's thick, jointed, fibrous stalks' internodes. Sugar cane in its raw state can be eaten by removing the outer layer and masticating the interior wet mass to extract the juice. The sugar cane is cold-pressed to produce sugar cane juice (guarapo). The glycemic index of sugar cane juice is lower than that of refined sugar cane.

Unrefined sugar is a healthy alternative to refined sugar and non-caloric artificial sweeteners (NAS). Refined sugar is an empty-calorie product that can be harmful to your health if ingested in significant quantities. According to a randomized study, NAS (saccharin, sucralose, aspartame, and acesulfame potassium) may cause obesity-related metabolic alterations by affecting the gut bacteria's function that colonizes the gut.[56] Noncentrifugal sugar (NCS) is the technical name for unprocessed raw sugar. This product has not been refined, so it still includes all the nutrients found in molasses.

The main ingredient in NCS is sucrose, which accounts for almost 80 percent of the total carbohydrate content (90 percent.) Calcium, potassium, sodium, chloride, and phosphates are all found in NCS. Iron, zinc, magnesium, copper, cobalt, nickel, and chromium are critical nutrients in NCS. The World Customs Organization defines NCS as "cane sugar produced without centrifugation." The product comprises only natural anhedral microcrystals of irregular shape, barely apparent to the human eye, surrounded by molasses residues and other sugar cane nutritious constituents.

Sugar that has been refined in a highly industrialized process may pose a health risk depending on how much of it you consume. Sugar, like wheat, is refined, and all its vitamins and nutrients are removed. The American Heart Association recommends no more than 9 teaspoons (36 grams) of added sugar per day for men. The figure for women is lower: 6 teaspoons (25 grams) per day and less than 24 grams for children under 18 years.[57] We consumed an average of 25 U.S. teaspoons every day or around four times more than is recommended. Refined sugar consumption has risen in the previous 60 years, to the point that 80 percent of packaged foods in a supermarket contain refined sugars. Refined sugar, whether brown or white, is dangerous to your health at that level of consumption.

The sugar industry has powerful lobbyists in Washington, DC, which thwarts any efforts to raise public awareness of sugar's harmful impacts on our health. So far, they've been able to block all attempts to regulate sugar. For example, the FDA has not been able to add the percentage of the recommended daily allowance of sugar on any food labels due to political contributions. Another reason why we can no longer trust the FDA.

§ §

B.3. Industrialized Vegetable Oils

Crisco shortening, a trans-fat produced from cottonseeds, was launched by Procter & Gamble in 1911. P&G marketed the product as a healthier alternative to lard, tallow, or butter, which were the most common natural cooking fats at the time. Crisco is deficient in the nutrients found in butterfat and other natural fats; indeed, all vegetable oils are deficient in these elements.[5]

Cottonseed oil was initially utilized as a lubricant for mechanical connections. Producing more oil than there was a demand for, vegetable oil makers advertised it as a healthier cooking alternative to natural fats: P&G was the first to do so with Crisco oil. Have you seen photos of vegetable oil refineries, by the way? Petroleum refineries in northern New Jersey, southern Texas, and southern California resemble them. During and after the saturated fat dispute in the 1970s, the use of vegetable oils skyrocketed. They've become an indisputable mainstay of ultraprocessed foods in American kitchens and restaurants, and they're slowly killing us.

The increased consumption of vegetable oils is correlated with the increased rate of heart disease deaths. In 1900 we consumed 2 grams of vegetable oil per capita per day, but by 2019, we consumed 800 grams per capita per day.[62] Today, there are more heart disease deaths than in the first half of the twentieth century. Omega-

6 fats are abundant in vegetable oils, and we consume far more omega-6 fats in our diet than is appropriate for our bodies. In 2010 we ingested 30 grams of omega-6 fats, a 15-fold increase over the prior 50 years, yet the consumption of omega-3 fats remained steady. Vegetable oils raise insulin levels and produce type 2 diabetes in a short period. Vegetable oils, like refined sugar, can cause fatty liver after 30 weeks of continuous consumption.[63] Vegetable oils and trans fats are found to be significant contributors to obesity and heart disease in obesity studies.

Obese persons in the United States have more omega-6 fats in their blood than people in other countries. Normal-weight Americans are unusual because their blood contains high quantities of omega-3 fats and low levels of omega-6 fats. The typical ratio of omega-6 to omega-3 fats in Americans is more than five times higher than in Europeans or Japanese people, according to Dr. Will Lassek.[11]

The industrial-era vegetable oils harmful to your health are canola, soy, sunflower, cottonseed, grapeseed, corn, safflower, and non-butter spreads (including margarine, mayonnaise, and salad dressing), to name a few.[60] According to research, palm oil is not a suitable substitute for partly hydrogenated fats (trans fats) because it causes detrimental changes in LDL and apolipoprotein B blood concentrations, much like a trans-fat.[66] These oils are poisonous due to the way they are processed, not because they are toxic at the source. All these PUFA oils go through a similar process. To remove the oil from the grain or seed, the manufacturer uses solvent extraction. Hexane, a derivative of petrochemicals like gasoline or diesel, is used as a solvent. Because the oil is not edible at this stage of the process and is highly hazardous, they must remove the solvent using heat and steam once the extraction is complete. The next stage is to purify it, which entails getting rid of the hexane. To finish the procedure, they must degum, neutralize, bleach, deodorize, winterize, and dewax it. Is this the type of oil you'd like to consume? PUFA oils are highly unstable, and the worst part is that they combine with oxygen to form reactive oxygen species, which are extremely harmful to human tissues. PUFAs increase insulin resistance, spike glucose to dangerously high levels, and cause chronic low-grade inflammation linked to degenerative diseases.[63, 67]

The healthy traditional fats are some of the best foods you can cook with and are natural. Animal fats (lard, tallow, dairy ghee, and dairy butter) and cold press extra virgin olive or avocado oil are also two healthy options.[60] Like extra virgin olive oil, edible unrefined cold-pressed avocado oil keeps the flavor and color qualities of the fruit flesh. Avocado oil has a comparable fat composition to olive oil. When avocado oil is refined, it is heated, and some of the nutritional benefits present in unrefined avocado oil are lost. Because of the color of the fruit, unrefined cold-pressed olive and avocado oil are green. They turn yellowish or amber in color after being purified and heated. The process of cooking raises the smoke point [8] of the oil. Although avocado oil is beneficial, there hasn't been enough long-term human research to see any adverse health impacts. Dr. Esselstyn advises against consuming oils if you have a cardiac condition.[17] Dairy ghee has a high smoke point and can be used for frying.

Vegetable oils are hydrogenated or partially hydrogenated fatty acids (trans fats), also called polyunsaturated fats (PUFAs). They have been found to clog arteries, which is why cardiovascular disease is on the rise. Erectile dysfunction (ED) is one of the first signs in men that their arteries are not functioning properly. The incidence of ED has risen considerably in recent years, and it could represent the proverbial canary in the coal mine, signaling that the arteries are becoming clogged. The heart's coronary artery could be next.[60] See Appendix C, *Government in the Public Interest?* For the latest government ruling on trans-fats.

§ §

---

[8] The temperature at which fats in cooking oils begin to degrade and produce smoke as the oil is heated. When oil reaches the temperature at which it begins to smoke, it undergoes a chemical breakdown, resulting in the emission of a gas and other pollutants. Because of this chemical breakdown, the oil may have an unpleasant taste.

B.4. Conclusion

The U.S. government and medical organization bureaucrats have confirmed 155-year-old common wisdom that a high-carbohydrate diet high in sugar causes obesity and associated diseases.

If the Senate Select Committee, which published the dietary guidelines in 1977, had read a document written in 1863, the country could have avoided a lot of suffering. William Banting wrote about his weight-loss challenges in that year. He struggled to lose weight despite eating less and exercising more, and he was always hungry. His dissatisfaction drove him to seek diet guidance from Dr. William Harvey. Mr. Banting chose to follow Dr. Harvey's advice and cut out carbohydrates, bread, refined grains, sugar, milk, alcohol, and starch (root vegetables and rice) from his diet. Banting shed 46 pounds in a year by eating three meals a day of fish, pork, and chicken, and many of his diseases disappeared. At the time, his book was a best-seller, and it is still in print today.[152] Books by Nina Teicholz and Gary Taubes provide a detailed account of Banting's fascinating story.[5, 32]

§ §

APPENDIX C.

GOVERNMENT IN THE PUBLIC INTEREST?

The United States Constitution proclaims that the government exists to serve the people. So why hasn't the government declared ultraprocessed foods to be dangerous to humans? We must wonder why our government takes such a long time to respond to public health crises. We recognize that corporations have the right to be heard in our democracy. But when political campaign contributions and lobbyist tactics abuse that right while the general public suffers, it's time to speak up. Food companies should not be allowed to add chemicals into our food supply unless there is a process to test such chemicals on animals and humans before releasing them into our food. It should be analogous to how new pharmaceutical medications get approved. Let us look at our slow government in action.

§ §

C.1. Asbestos

In 1931, the British Inspector of Factories issued a report to the British Parliament that resulted in the first regulation of the asbestos sector in the United Kingdom. The US government created regulations in 1943 to safeguard the navy shipyard personnel from asbestos dust, but it took another three decades for the government to enforce those standards. The United States is one of the few developed countries that has not eliminated asbestos use altogether.[153]

Executives in the asbestos sector understood that their product was hazardous to humans. When litigants sued the firms for asbestos-related ailments in the late 1970s, it came to the surface. Government authorities in the United States were negligent in their duty; they were aware that asbestos was dangerous to humans but did nothing to prohibit firms from selling it.[153] Finally, in 2020, a United States House of Representatives committee decided unanimously to submit a bill banning the use of asbestos to the House floor for a vote. It has not been debated on the floor yet. Although the United States is getting closer to outlawing asbestos, the United Kingdom has been asbestos-free for nearly a century. Other countries have either outright banned asbestos or enacted rigorous legislation to safeguard their citizens from it. The United States has not prohibited asbestos, and the regulations that have been enacted are inadequate.[153] Now Congress will try one more time.

§ §

C.2. Lead Paint

Lead is a neurotoxin that damages the neurological system, stunts children's growth, damages the kidneys, and delays brain development. Lead poisoning can be fatal in high doses. Under German health legislation, women and children were forbidden from working in factories that handled lead paint as early as 1886. Benjamin Franklin wrote a letter to a friend in 1786, warning him of the dangers of lead paints, which he thought were well known.[154] In an unprecedented step by a corporation, Sherwin-Williams revealed the dangers of lead paint in a July 1904 company publication, stating that a French expert had considered lead paint "poisonous to a significant degree, both for the employees and for the inhabitants of a house painted with lead colors."

When preventive actions were needed in the past, responses to lead-based paint were reactive. The government concentrated on youngsters getting lead poisoning from eating paint chips, ignoring lead-contaminated dust and dirt. The danger of lead dust is that it can be accidentally inhaled. Lead-based paint regulation was implemented in several areas as early as the 1950s. There was little understanding of the hazards of lead dust during this time. Our government did not prohibit the use of lead in the paint until 1978.

Early in the twentieth century, foreign countries outlawed the use of lead in paints. It took the US government 74 years to ban lead paints even when a major US firm admitted that its paints contained lead and were dangerous to the public 74 years earlier.

§ §

C.3. Leaded Gasoline

The Ethyl Gasoline Corporation was founded in 1924 by General Motors and the Standard Oil Company (Exxon) to develop and distribute tetraethyl lead (TEL), a lead additive to gasoline, to increase the octane level. However, the new facility was beset by cases of lead poisoning, hallucinations, insanity, and five deaths in the first two months of operation in 1924. State authorities shot down the new facility in New Jersey.[155]

The Clean Air Act is a federal statute in the United States that regulates national air pollution. It was first enacted in 1963, and it has been revised several times since then. The United States Congress considerably enlarged the federal obligation in the Clean Air Amendments of 1970, requiring extensive federal and state industrial and mobile sources restrictions. The bill established the National Emissions Standards for Hazardous Air Pollutants and bolstered government enforcement authorities to pursue aggressive air pollution reduction targets. The Environmental Protection Agency (EPA) was established in 1970 and mandated to control substances that damage human health. The EPA ordered a gradual reduction in lead levels in all gasoline grades in 1973.[155]

The Environmental Protection Agency (EPA) mandated that at least one grade of unleaded gasoline be compatible with 1975 cars in 1974. Catalytic converters were being put on cars, and lead was causing damage to the catalytic converters used to reduce exhaust emissions in these new vehicles. The Environmental Protection Agency (EPA) banned leaded gasoline for on-road cars in 1996. (Leaded gasoline sales were down to 0.6 percent by 1996). We've known for 72 years that lead in gasoline is harmful to humans, but it's taken that long for the government to act. The government gesture was meaningless since almost no one was buying leaded gasoline at the time. Some aircraft fuels still include the lead component.

§ §

C.4. Cigarette Smoking and Vaping

The British Medical Journal released an article in September 1950 associating smoking with lung cancer and heart disease.[156] Despite this warning, people continued to smoke due to nicotine addiction. Smoking is harmful to nearly every organ in the body and is a leading cause of heart attacks, strokes, and cancer. The tobacco industry has been staunchly opposed to the implementation of cigarette warning labels. As we all know, tobacco executives lied to Congress about the dangers of cigarette smoking and what they knew about them. The United States government ultimately required a warning from the surgeon general on cigarette packs in 1966; nevertheless, the warning was weak and ambiguous. It had been 16 years since the British journal article. After the states successfully sued the tobacco firms for health-related charges, it took another 25 years to issue a harsher warning.

Vaping is the most recent version of smoking. The Centers for Disease Control and Prevention strongly linked an outbreak of severe vaping lung ailments in the United States in 2019 and to vitamin E acetate in 2020. E-cigarettes emit the same number of particles into the air as traditional cigarettes. According to a study published in 2020, e-cigarettes raise the risk of asthma by 40 percent and chronic obstructive pulmonary disease by 50 percent. Many e-cigarettes include nicotine, which has been linked to severe health problems, and e-cigarette aerosols can contain harmful chemicals. Cancer-causing substances and microscopic particles that penetrate deep into the lungs are among them.[81] How long will it take this time to get a strong warning label from the surgeon general on every vaping product?

§ §

C.5. Trans Fats

Many countries have passed legislation aimed at limiting fat-containing trans fatty acids (vegetable oils). Scientists in the field of lipid studies first raised the alarm in 1956—numerous researches stating that considerable negative health impacts from trans fats prompted these regulations. Trans fats are thought to play a role in various disorders, including cardiovascular disease, diabetes, and cancer. Trans fats included in vegetable oils increase the risk of heart disease, the leading cause of death among adults in the United States. The more vegetable oil with trans fats you consume, the higher your risk of heart and blood vessel disease.[157]

Trans fats have been linked to a considerable increase in coronary artery disease since 1956, according to scientific research. However, the concerns had been ignored for six decades. Finally, the FDA determined in 2015 that partly hydrogenated oils (PHOs) are not Generally Recognized as Safe (GRAS). The compliance date to stop manufacturing foods with PHOs had been extended to June 2019 to give time for reformulation. These products will go through distribution until 2021. PHOs were found to be responsible for hundreds of thousands of heart attack deaths, prompting this action.

It had been 60 years since the lipid scientists had raised the alarm. The Food and Drug Administration has allowed food makers six years to remove the chemical from the food supply. Despite this, the government has not informed the public about PHOs' hazards so that people can avoid purchasing these food products. In the meantime, the estimated 100,000 fatalities caused by trans-fats per year will continue. According to a randomized study, a 2 percent increase in trans-fat calories doubles the risk of heart disease.[14, 82, 148] The FDA's action is a tacit admission that this chemical is a toxin and that it has taken too long to eliminate its usage in our food supply. Food businesses should be held accountable for the pain and deaths caused by their hazardous products, which have resulted in hundreds of thousands of deaths.

§ §

C.6. Conclusions

These are only a few of the most egregious examples of the US government's failure to act in the public interest.

- Is the ultraprocessed food sector going to be the same? Over the last 50 years, as our intake of ultraprocessed foods has climbed, so has the prevalence of metabolic syndrome disorders. How much longer must we wait for, at the very least, to get a warning label on ultraprocessed foods and sugary beverages?
- Why can't the maximum quantity of refined sugar recommended per day be listed on nutritional labels of food packages? Or a percentage of the daily value? Why is the FDA not doing it?
- What about PUFAs (polyunsaturated fatty acids)? When will we have at least a warning label that says they could be harmful to our health, even for oils with less than .5 per serving?
- The government should require the food sector to reformulate its processed food products to remove harmful components in an ideal world. If they do not, the people will be forced to take health-related action in spite of their government.

- Why do foreign governments take actions to protect the health of their citizens earlier, in many cases decades, than our government?

Draw your own conclusions.

§ §

APPENDIX D.

A BRIEFING ON THE METABOLIC SYNDROME

D.1. The Significance of the Metabolic Syndrome

In this Appendix, we shall explain a significant medical problem in the United States that has turned into a self-inflicted health disaster. The most severe disease is metabolic syndrome, which refers to a group of chronic disorders that have developed in an otherwise healthy environment as a result of the Western diet.[29] Its symptoms can be avoided and, in most cases, reversed with healthy natural nutrition. We'll concentrate on type 2 diabetes, the most common metabolic syndrome disease and seems to promote other chronic diseases.

If you are interested in this subject and want more in-depth knowledge, we recommend the books by Dr. Jason Fung, *The Diabetes Code*,[37] and Dr. Robert Lustig, *Fat Chance*.[6]

§ §

D.2. Metabolic Syndrome: Type 2 Diabetes as the Sentinel Disease

Many people in the United States died from cardiovascular disease throughout the 1940s, 50s, and 60s. High cholesterol levels in the arteries, which led to heart attacks and strokes, were blamed on saturated fat found in meats and dairy foods. Refined carbohydrates, such as those found in bread, pasta, rice, and sugar, gained a foothold in the food discussion in the 1970s. The low-fat, high-carbohydrate diet was born when they were pushed as healthier options in the government's dietary guidelines of 1977.

Over the last 20 years, randomized research trials have debunked the myth that saturated fat consumption causes high cholesterol or cardiovascular disease. We've been terrified of natural foods like meats and dairy foods because of saturated fat for the previous 50 years. Yet, saturated fat is actually beneficial and may help prevent some chronic diseases.[5, 9, 148] We've cut saturated fat consumption to the government's recommended level, but cardiovascular death rates are now higher than they were in the 1950s and 1960s. In addition, we have a slew of new chronic illnesses by adopting the low-fat/high-carb diet, labeled as the *metabolic syndrome.*

Metabolism: "The sum of the processes of protoplasm (proteins and water) buildup and destruction, precisely: the chemical changes in living cells that generate energy for essential processes and activities while also assimilating new material."[158]

Syndrome: "A cluster of disease-related signs and symptoms that appear simultaneously and indicate a particular anomaly or condition."[158]

The medical establishment has defined *metabolic syndrome* phenomenologically, meaning with measurements and parameters shown in the figure below. The problem with using measurements is that they are imprecise. If they are a few points over or under "normal," what does that mean? No one can tell you for sure. Remember that Dr. Robert Lustig does not think specific measurements are the right way to define metabolic syndrome. The syndrome should be defined mechanistically as insulin resistance.[29]

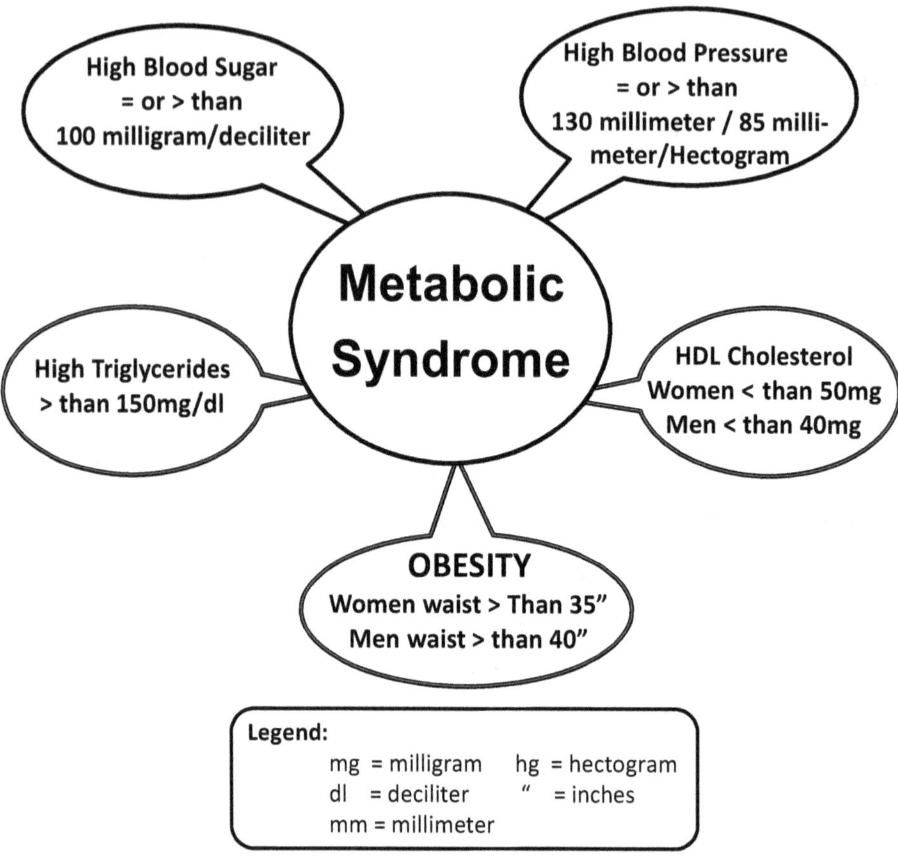

Figure 2. Metabolic syndrome is a dangerous disorder that many individuals are unaware of until it is too late. According to the American Heart Association, the components depicted in the diagram are the ones most typically associated with metabolic syndrome. The condition is identified when three of the five risk factors are present.[159]

High blood pressure, elevated blood sugar (pre-diabetes), low levels of good cholesterol (high-density lipids [HDLs]), high triglyceride levels, and a big waist circumference (obesity) are common symptoms of the metabolic syndrome, as shown in figure 2. An underlying bodily disorder of energy utilization and storage is assumed to be the cause of the syndrome.[37]

According to Dr. Robert Lustig, there are three different manifestations of metabolic syndrome:[29]

(1) *Subcutaneous fat, which is the fat below the waist (hips, legs, buttocks) found in obese persons and which everyone believes is the source of the problem*

(2) *Visceral fat (beer belly), or fat that has accumulated in the stomach area, necessitates a CT scan to evaluate the fat that has accumulated in the internal organs*

(3) *Fatty liver (liver fat) is caused by too much fructose (sugar) being processed in the liver over time*

Many doctors blame obesity for type 2 diabetes and metabolic syndrome. We need to reframe the discussion, according to Dr. Robert Lustig. Obesity, he believes, is not the cause of the metabolic syndrome but rather a consequence of it. Obesity, he believes, is a "red herring" that only serves to confuse the underlying issue.[29] Metabolic syndrome can affect anyone, regardless of weight.[13]

Obesity increases at a global rate of 2.78 percent per year, whereas diabetes rises at 4.07 percent. If obesity is the problem, why is diabetes growing faster than obesity (almost twice as fast)?[14] According to what we learned, most Cubans were normal-weight, and obesity was not a factor in their health crisis. Despite this, high levels of metabolic syndrome existed before the 1990s health crisis, supporting Dr. Lustig's hypothesis.

Metabolic syndrome sick is strongly linked to insulin resistance, according to medical professionals. When it comes to insulin resistance, where does it come from? According to medical research, the amount of fat in the liver influences insulin dynamics. A fatty liver is a symptom of metabolic syndrome, a risk factor for type 2 diabetes. The liver metabolizes four chemicals that, if taken in excess and frequently, may cause fatty liver disease:

- Trans fats (hydrogenated vegetable oils)
- Branched-chain amino acids (found in protein-powered, corn-fed beef and corn-fed chicken). Note that pasture-raised beef and chicken are healthier
- Alcohol
- Sugar in any form, including high-fructose corn syrup (HFCS); sugar is the most harmful because of the amount we consume on a daily basis and the way our bodies metabolize it.[160]

Because of its chemistry, sugar must be addressed while discussing metabolic syndrome. Sucrose is a sugar that is half glucose and half fructose. Glucose is easily absorbed throughout the body, whereas fructose is sent immediately to the liver, the only organ that can metabolize fructose. Excess fructose in the liver is converted to fat.[159]

Nonalcoholic fatty liver disease (NAFLD) and alcoholic fatty liver disease (AFLD) are the two most common kinds of fatty liver disease. Alcohol is only metabolized in the liver, and excessive alcohol drinking causes cirrhosis, a fatty liver disease. NAFLD is a relatively new and rapidly spreading disorder caused by the liver's inability to process significant fructose (sugar) levels. Sugar (fructose) accumulates in the liver as fat. Insulin resistance induces fat infiltration and inflammation in the liver, resulting in NAFLD. Sugar contains fructose, which has the same effect on the liver as alcohol. The liver is the only organ capable of breaking down fructose. Insulin does not regulate fructose.[6]

Several other factors influence metabolic syndrome. The Western diet plays a significant role, according to research, because of the increased consumption of ultraprocessed fast food, which is not biochemically suited to humans.[6, 8, 51] metabolic syndrome affects 60 percent of the US population over the age of 50. When it comes to that population, women have a higher prevalence of the syndrome than men. Type 2 diabetes, according to Dr. Jason Fung, is unlike any other disease physicians have encountered. It has the capacity to decimate our bodies. Diabetes affects nearly every organ system in the body.[37]

§ §

D.3. Insulin: Encouraging Fat Storage

Insulin is a natural hormone that transports glucose throughout the body to provide energy to cells and muscles. The pancreas produces insulin. Obesity is mainly caused by an excess of insulin in the body. Fats, proteins, and carbohydrates are the three essential elements of our food, and they are processed differently by our digestive system. Fats are broken down into fatty acids, proteins are broken down into amino acids, and carbohydrates are broken down into sugars.[7, 24]

One of insulin's most important functions is to allow glucose (sugar) to enter cells and generate energy.[37] Fatty acids are vital structural components of cells and critical nutritional fuels for humans. Fatty acids are taken directly into the bloodstream by the body. Fatty acids do not alter insulin levels because they bypass the liver, so a high-fat, low-carb diet is suggested for type 2 diabetes.[94] Because of its refined carbohydrates, a slice of white bread, for example, will trigger a glucose spike. Because of the butterfat, the spike decreases if you spread dairy butter on the piece of bread. People who are prediabetic or have type 2 diabetes should not begin eating slices of bread with butter since the butter lessens but does not eliminate the spike.

Food energy is stored in the adipose tissue as body fat, while excess glucose is stored as glycogen (starch) in the liver. The amount of glycogen that the liver can store is restricted. When the liver is full, the excess glycogen is converted to fat through a process known as *de novo lipogenesis*.[37] De novo lipogenesis is a complex, tightly regulated metabolic system in which carbohydrates in the bloodstream are converted to fatty acids, then used to make triglycerides for energy storage. Carbohydrates, like fructose, move straight to the liver, where they are metabolized and turned into fat. When the liver is overloaded with fat, the mitochondria are overwhelmed, leading to fatty liver and insulin resistance.[50]

When insulin is blocked from penetrating the cells, the pancreas compensates by producing more insulin, resulting in *hyperinsulinemia*.[37] This illness causes excessive insulin levels in the blood, which leads to weight gain. According to Dr. Fung, it's a two-step process in which our bodies use the energy they need and store the rest for later use. Glycogen is a kind of glucose that humans use to store energy. Glycogen is predominantly produced and stored in the liver and skeletal muscle cells. We aggravate these processes by eating 6 to 10 times every day, generating a constant supply of insulin, and storing the excess. Our several daily meal sessions frequently cause the fat buildup.[95] If insulin levels remain high, the body is constantly signaled to store food energy as body fat leading to obesity.

§ §

D.4. Insulin Resistance: The Culprit

Insulin resistance is a disease-related condition in which cells do not respond appropriately to the hormone insulin. Obesity is thought to come before type 2 diabetes, according to conventional wisdom. The difficulty with that assumption is that while millions of obese people do not have type 2 diabetes, millions of persons of normal weight do (we discussed this earlier in the section on metabolic syndrome).[29] Our bodies acquire resistance to any substance that makes us unstable, according to Dr. Jason Fung. The body works towards homeostasis or equilibrium. When the pancreas produces too much insulin, the body reacts by fighting the extra insulin; however, the excess insulin must be stored, and it is stored as fat in our cells.

Sugar, also known as sucrose, is a carbohydrate that contains 50 percent glucose and 50 percent fructose. A 150-pound woman is given 6 U.S. teaspoonfuls of sugar, of which 3 teaspoons are glucose, which is metabolized throughout the body. The remaining 3 teaspoons of fructose are directly digested in the 4- or 5-pound liver. Because fructose is stored in the liver as glycogen (a type of starch), it overwhelms the organ. It turns to fat, signaling the start of a fatty liver and insulin resistance.

The pancreas produces insulin in reaction to carbohydrates in the diet. Insulin resistance necessitates the use of more insulin to transfer glucose into our cells. Obesity, a sedentary lifestyle, a family history of diabetes, high blood pressure, and certain medications are common risk factors for insulin resistance. Insulin resistance is a crucial indicator of metabolic syndrome. Hyperinsulinemia is a condition caused by elevated insulin levels. The available medications on the market only treat the symptoms of hyperinsulinemia, not the underlying cause of insulin resistance. Obesity is a common side effect of this illness, and obesity and type 2 diabetes are both indications of hyperinsulinemia.[37]

Dietary choices influence insulin resistance. Insulin resistance has been linked to foods that are high in sugar (carbohydrates) and have high glycemic indices (GI), as well as those that are high in fructose, low in omega-3 fats and fiber, and those that are hyperpalatable (sweetened with sugar). Eating items fried in vegetable oils can produce fatty liver in a short period. Due to the high content of omega-6 fats, vegetable oils can also cause inflammation and cardiovascular diseases. As we now know, a fatty liver plays a crucial role in the development of insulin resistance.

One of the causes of insulin resistance happens when your liver retains fat, and your pancreas' ability to release insulin weakens over time, resulting in type 2 diabetes. So when physicians talk about too much sugar and type 2 diabetes, they are simply talking about blood sugar (glucose). Insulin resistance is diagnosed using fasting blood glucose meters and A1C blood sugar measurements. When our blood sugar levels are high, our bodies respond by producing more insulin, and if we don't change our diet, our bodies will eventually develop insulin resistance. As a result, when you develop insulin resistance, your cells no longer require all the glucose. The extra energy (glucose) that your body does not need is stored in your skin cells. It starts with high blood sugar caused by eating foods with high carbohydrates and a high glycemic index (GI).

We have referred to foods with a high glycemic index (GI). The GI measures how quickly a carbohydrate is absorbed and how quickly blood sugar levels rise. Because there is another critical factor: glycemic load (GL). The GL accounts for how much carbs are present in the food and how much each gram of carb raises blood glucose levels. A raw carrot, for example, has a GI of 91, which means it will cause your blood sugar to increase, but when you look at the GL, you'll notice that it is just 1 or very low. Because the fiber in the carrot is high, the GL is just 1, indicating that the carrot fiber will feed your biome and slow the sugar released while having almost no effect on your blood sugar.

It's crucial to think about both the glycemic load and the glycemic index. Corn, for example, has a GI of 55, which is moderate, and a GL of 62, which is exceptionally high and will dangerously spike your blood sugar. You can calculate the glycemic load fairly quickly. The formula is:

GL = (GI x the amount of carbohydrate) divided by 100

(For example, an apple; GI 40 X carbs 15 / 100 = 6)

The impact on our liver is a part of the biochemistry effect. When the liver becomes overburdened with fructose, the liver becomes overwhelmed, and a fatty liver develops. Insulin resistance, according to traditional medicine, has no cure. What physicians mean is that a pill or an injection will not cure it. Current medications exacerbate the problem since they only address one cause: high blood sugar (glucose). Therefore, they try to lower blood sugar, but not insulin levels, and only excess insulin can create insulin resistance.

However, let us look at the real issue: your body has three areas that react to food: blood sugar (glucose), insulin (a hormone), and cells (adipocytes or fat cells composed of adipose tissue, specialized in storing energy as fat). Essentially, blood glucose is the energy that the insulin hormone transports to our cells throughout the body. Insulin becomes resistant when it is overwhelmed by glucose, and the pancreas produces more insulin. Therefore, too much insulin stimulates insulin resistance. It's just another example of why calorie counting is useless in the fight against insulin resistance. Carbohydrates with a high GI or high GL, not calorie intake, are the danger. Let us look at the metrics the physicians use:

Description	**Normal**	**Disease**
1. Glucose	70-100 mg/dl	>125
2. AIC	4.0-5.6 percent	>6.5
3. Insulin	2.6-25	>>
4. HOMA-IR*	0.5-1.5	$\frac{\text{Glucose X Insulin}}{405}$

* Homeostatic model assessment of insulin resistance

Physicians use items 1 and 2 to determine if you have type 2 diabetes. Because you don't develop diabetes overnight, they should also look at insulin level and HOMA-IR. Becoming insulin-resistant is a long process; you'll need to look at components 3 and 4 to figure out where you are in terms of insulin resistance. You become pre-diabetic; when your glucose is somewhat higher than 100, and when your glucose is above 125, and your A1C is 6.6, you have type 2 diabetes. The glucose rises to the disease level only when you are already pre-diabetic or have type 2 diabetes.[37] You should ask your doctor to check your insulin hormone level; if it is rapidly rising, even if it is below 25, it means you will become insulin resistant very soon.

§ §

D.5. Diabetes (Type 2 Diabetes): A World Pandemic?

Diabetes mellitus is the medical term for elevated blood sugar. Type 2 diabetes differs from type 1 diabetes in several ways. Type 2 diabetes, according to Dr. Jason Fung, is the most deadly medical condition associated with metabolic syndrome.[37]

For thousands of years, diabetes has been recognized. The ancient Egyptians detected diabetes in patients who urinated frequently. The term diabetes was coined by the ancient Greeks (excessive urination). The ailment was known as "sweet urine" in ancient China. In traditional Chinese medicine, doctors advised patients to avoid sweet foods like honey and instead use an extract from the monk fruit as a sweetener that would not create sweet urine (i.e., it did not raise blood sugar levels).

As we previously said, type 2 diabetes is increasing at nearly twice the rate of obesity. Type 2 diabetes affected 151 million persons globally in 2000. Based on that percentage, it was predicted that by 2010, 221 million individuals worldwide would have type 2 diabetes, a 46 percent increase at a projected yearly rate of 3.88 percent. In 2010, the actual number was 285 million individuals globally, growing at a 6.55 percent annual rate, or nearly double what was predicted in 2000. By 2014, that number had risen to 422 million at a yearly pace of 10.3 percent, and it is still growing.[1] Type 2 diabetes is expected to increase by 40 percent in the United States and 85 percent in China during the next 30 years. Also, in the next 30 years, the global growth rate is expected to be 38 percent.

This disease affects more individuals around the world than COVID-19, which has been labeled a pandemic. Obesity has been treated with high-carbohydrate, low-fat, and low-calorie diets, yet the condition persists. Because what we're doing is not working, we need to take a completely different approach. We are in the midst of a global pandemic that has the potential to destroy every country's healthcare system. Metabolic syndrome disease is responsible for 75 percent of healthcare costs in the United States and is growing.[159]

The traditional approach for treatment for type 2 diabetes has not worked. We began giving the patient insulin, which exacerbated the situation because insulin resistance is one of the most common symptoms. People gained more weight as a result of the increased insulin; consequently, we worsened rather than alleviated the problem. We were then sold on the idea that if we ate fewer calories and did more activity to burn them off, we would lose weight and reduce our diabetes.

Because it is not a physiological model, the calorie-in, calorie-out diet has failed. Dietitians use calories to calculate the intake necessary to reduce our weight. The problem with that approach is that they use a physics model; our bodies do not have a system to measure calories.[161] Calorie counting does not work in your body because when you reduce your caloric intake by eating less, your body adapts by slowing down your metabolism, which means you do not lose much weight and are constantly hungry.

Our dietary habits are also a problem. We ate three times a day in the early twentieth century, but we began to eat 6 to 10 times a day by the second half of the century. We eat the customary three meals a day and a coffee break with pastries in the middle of the morning, a sweet or fried snack in the middle of the afternoon, and one or two more snacks at night. The snacks mainly are ultraprocessed items with a lot of sugar and vegetable oils. Our metabolism never stops working because we've been eating more frequently. Obesity, according to Dr. Fung, is caused by a hormonal imbalance rather than a calorie imbalance. “Excess insulin, a hormone, is the fundamental hormonal problem in undesired weight gain.”[37] Thus, type 2 diabetes is a disease of insulin imbalance rather than a caloric imbalance.

§ §

D.6. Is Type 2 Diabetes Reversible?

Type 2 diabetes, according to Dr. Jason Fung, is a treatable dietary and lifestyle disorder. The notion has been proven in morbidly obese persons who underwent bariatric surgery (severe weight loss surgery). Diabetes was eliminated in just a few weeks in these people.[24] It has been proven time and time again with various types of weight-loss surgery. The point is that type 2 diabetes is a disease that can be reversed.

The medical community classifies type 2 diabetes as a chronic, progressive condition that affects people for the rest of their lives; sadly, there is no cure.[37] Standard drugs and lifestyle changes (low-fat, low-calorie diets) do not work for the morbidly obese. Hence surgery is recommended. According to data, it was recognized as early as the 1990s, but it took another 26 years, until 2016, for the recommendation to switch from diet to surgery. The technique was made available as a primary therapy option for people with type 2 diabetes and a BMI of 40 or higher.[37]

A ketogenic diet, according to Drs. Eric Westman, Stephen Phinney, and Jeff Volek's studies can reverse or significantly reduce type 2 diabetes.[94] Obesity and type 2 diabetes are on the rise due to an increase in refined carbohydrate consumption. Apart from the few carbs in green leafy vegetables, the keto diet eliminates refined carbohydrates and reduces carbohydrates in general. It is misleading to argue that a particular diet is beneficial or bad for the overall population. As suggested in Chapter 12, we are all different physiologically, and some foods affect us differently. As a result, we recommend a personalized diet based on cutting-edge techniques for those people with underlying medical conditions like metabolic syndrome.

We also know that intermittent fasting reduces weight, reverses type 2 diabetes, and lowers high blood pressure, as we demonstrated in Chapter 7, "A time to eat and a time not to eat." From all the data, we can safely argue that type 2 diabetes is reversible and does not have to be with you for the rest of your life.

§ §

D.7. The New Science of Autophagy: Regeneration

Autophagy is derived from the Greek words auto, which means "self," and phage, which means "to eat." As a result, autophagy means "self-eating." When researchers discovered that a cell could destroy its contents in the 1960s, they came up with this concept.

Dr. Yoshinori Ohsumi of Japan identified the mechanisms of autophagy in human cells in the 1990s. His findings ushered in a new way of thinking about how the human cell recycles its contents. He paved the way for a better understanding of autophagy's role in various physiological processes, such as starvation adaptation and infection response. Fasting, for example, causes a significant increase in autophagy. Fasting permits unwanted proteins to be destroyed and amino acids to be recycled more efficiently to produce proteins required for survival and new cell growth.[162] Ohsumi won the 2016 Nobel Prize for Physiology and Medicine for his work on autophagy.

What is the significance of this human mechanism? Autophagy is a highly controlled process in which your cells break down and eat their own components for nutrition. The procedure clears the body of dead cells. Fasting improves the function of the brain and other organs due to the chemical changes caused by autophagy. Although no studies have been conducted to determine the period of fasting required to start autophagy, the best estimations suggest that at least

36 hours of water-only fasting is required. Fasting not only helps to lessen type 2 diabetes, but it also helps to clear dead cells and recycle them so that your body can build new cells faster than normal processes.[162]

The human body is a marvelous biochemical construct that can restore itself. Fasting, according to Hippocrates, the father of medicine, helps the body repair itself.[24]

§ §

WHO WE ARE

As children of Cuban immigrants, our parents wanted to ensure that we were raised like normal American children. We grew up in typical American suburbia in close proximity to major cities. Growing up, we lived in various places across the country and learned about their distinct regional characteristics. As we finished our graduate degrees and settled into adulthood, we developed an interest in our past.

Our ancestors came from the Kingdom of Spain. In the 1880s, our great grandparents arrived in Cuba from northern Spain. On our father's side of the family, they were from Asturias, officially known as the Principality of Asturias, an autonomous region. Our mother's side of the family came from the Basque Country, an autonomous region in the Pyrenees Mountains.

Our mother was born in the Cuban city of Caibarien, whereas our father was born in Havana, Cuba's capital. When the communist took over Cuba, they emigrated to the United States, where we were born. Our family has a history of overcoming difficulties, adapting, and achieving in the face of adversity. Our parents instilled in us the drive to study and learn and the value of putting in the effort required to succeed.[163]

Emilio Collar, Jr., PhD

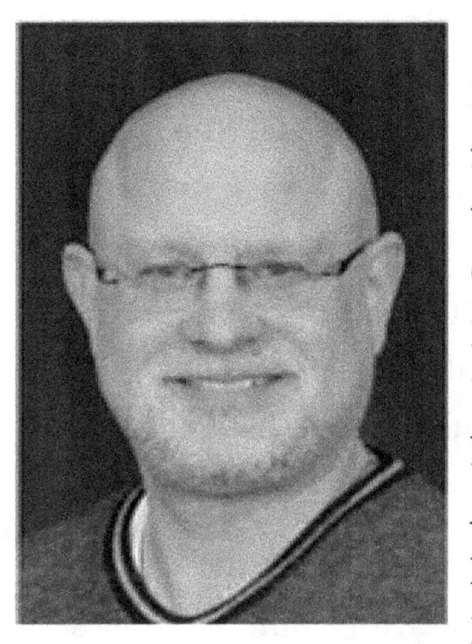

Dr. Emilio Collar earned his Doctorate in Information Systems from the Leeds School of Business at the University of Colorado, Boulder, Colorado; his Master of Science in Information Systems from Pace University, New York, New York; and his Bachelor of Business Administration from Pace University, New York, New York. He is currently a Professor of Management Information Systems at Western Connecticut State University, Danbury, Connecticut.

He is a KPMG Foundation Doctoral Scholar and a member of Beta Gamma Sigma.

Prior to his Ph.D., Dr. Collar has had various jobs and consulting engagements in large Corporations, including General Reinsurance Corp. and IBM. As an independent consultant, Dr. Collar has provided consulting services on software implementation of Oracle databases, Internet website development, e-Commerce applications, and Internet security and planning. Dr. Collar was also a technology consultant for the IBM Information Technology implementation at the 1998 Nagano Winter Olympic Games and

2000 Sydney Summer Olympic Games. He analyzed and documented the Information Technology deployment identifying the processes required for the deployment of the operation of the software applications.

Dr. Collar co-founded an organization called The International Group of E-business Research and Applications (TIGERA) and served as Vice President from 2006 to 2011. It provided a forum for scholars, professionals, students, and Government representatives to present their latest findings in e-Learning, e-Business, and e-Government research, applications, and the underlying technologies.

Dr. Collar has served as editing manager for the Journal of Computing and e-Systems, track chair for multiple topics at TIGERA, and as a guest or invited reviewer for various academic journals.

He has published papers in academic journals including *Cybernetics and Informatics, International Journal of Computer Science and Information Security, International Journal of Management Science and Business Administration, Journal of Management and Business Research, Journal of Systemics, European Business Review, and International Journal of Global Business and Competitiveness.*

Lisette Collar, RDMS

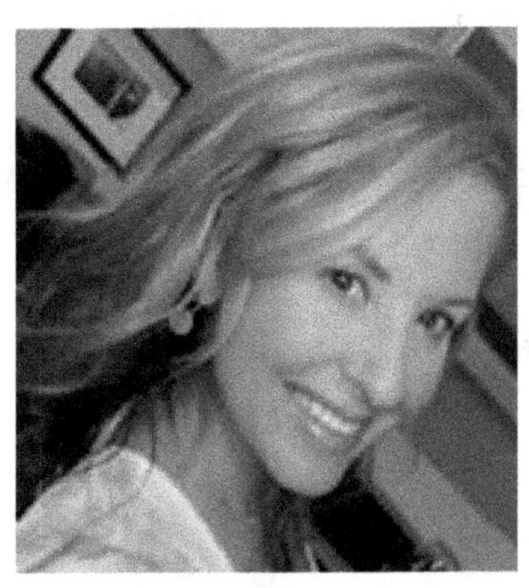

Ms. Collar earned a Graduate Diploma in Medical Informatics from the University of West Florida, Pensacola, Florida; a Bachelor of Arts Degree in Social Sciences from Washington State University, Pullman, Washington; and an Associate of Science in Diagnostic Medical Sonography from Sanford-Brown Institute, Ft. Lauderdale, Florida. She is a Registered Diagnostic Medical Sonographer with the American Registry for Diagnostic Medical Sonography (RDMS).

Ms. Collar has been a business consultant for various business organizations. She was a sonographer at renowned American hospitals, including Mount Sinai Medical Center, New York, New York, and a Clinical Specialist at Baptist Hospital, Miami, Florida. She has been an Adjunct Instructor of Sonography for various technical colleges in Florida.

A Diagnostic Medical Sonographer uses imaging equipment and soundwaves to form images of many parts of the body known as Ultrasound. Ultrasound is a non-invasive way to visualize internal organs. Sonographers play an essential role in conducting and interpreting imaging tests to aid the Radiologist in a patient's diagnosis. It requires extensive knowledge in anatomy and physiology, mathematics, and physics. Ms. Collar specialized in Abdomen, Small Parts, OB/GYN, Neuro, Vascular, and Breast. As a Clinical Specialist, she worked with Radiologists to create protocol procedures for the imaging department. She also worked at Level One Trauma facilities in the Emergency Room and performed ultrasound-guided procedures in the Operating Room.

****

ACKNOWLEDGMENTS

We want to thank our editor, Marjorie Toensing, for her extraordinary and thorough job and suggestions. She is everything we could hope for in an editor.

We thank you, Dr. Stuart Varden, for his review and valuable comments.

We also want to thank the authors and researchers we have used as references; this book is better because of their expertise and published works.

****

References

1. Lustig, R.H., *Fat Chance: Fructose 2.0 (Lecture).* 2013, YouTube: https://www.youtube.com/watch?v=ceFyF9px20Y.

2. Franco, M., et al., *Impact of Energy Intake, Physical Activity, and Population-wide Weight Loss on Cardiovascular Disease and Diabetes Mortality in Cuba, 1980–2005.* American Journal of Epidemiology., 2007. **Volume 166**(Issue 12): p. 1374–1380.

3. Franco, M., et al., *Population-wide weight loss and regain in relation to diabetes burden and cardiovascular mortality in Cuba1980-2010: Repeated cross-sectional surveys and ecological comparison of secular trends.* British Medical Journal, 2013: p. 2013: 346:f1515.

4. Peterson, P. *Why Are Americans Paying More for Healthcare?* https://www.pgpf.org/blog/2020/04/why-are-americans-paying-more-for-healthcare, 2020, Apr. 20.

5. Teicholz, N., *The Big Fat Surprise: Why Butter, Meat and Cheese Belong in a Healthy Diet.* 2015, Simon & Schuster. p. 497.

6. Lustig, R.H., *Fat Chance: Beating the Odds Against Sugar, Processed Food, Obesity, and Disease* 2012, Hudson Street Press - Penguin Group: Amazon.

7. Ludwig, D., *Always Hungry?: Conquer Cravings, Retrain Your Fat Cells, and Lose Weight Permanently.* 2016: Amazon.

8. Pollan, M., *In Defense of Food: An Eater's Manifesto.* 2009, Penguin Books. p. 268.

9. Taubes, G., *The Case for Keto: Rethinking Weight Control and the Science and Practice of Low-Carb/High-Fat Eating.* 2020, A. Knopf: Amazon.

10. Collins, S. *Hidden Dangers of Ultraprocessed Foods.* https://www.webmd.com/sonya-collins, 2020, Feb 21.

11. Lassek, W. *Why Are We Eating so Much More Than We Used to? How "bad" fats make us gain weight.* https://www.psychologytoday.com/us/blog/why-women-need-fat/201205/why-are-we-eating-so-much-more-we-used, 2012, May 11.

12. Schwarz, M. and M. Pollan, *In Defense of Food: An Eater's Manifesto (Documentary).* 2015, YouTube: https://www.youtube.com/watch?v=95mdAHDK_JM.

13. Lustig, R.M., *Metabolical: The Lure and the Lies of Processed Food, Nutrition, and Modern Medicine.* 2021, HarperCollins Publishers Australia Pty. Ltd.: Amazon.

14. Lustig, R.H., *Processed Food: An Experiment That Failed (Lecture).* 2017, YouTube: https://www.youtube.com/watch?v=pvgxNDuQ5DI.

15. History_Scope, *The Breakup of the Soviet Union Explained*, in *History Scope.* 2019, YouTube: https://www.youtube.com/watch?v=t2GmtBCVHzY.

16. Fulkerson, L., *Forks Over Knives (Documentary).* 2011, YouTube: https://www.youtube.com/watch?v=n1LUj3kxB9M.

17. EsselstynJr, C.B., *Prevent and Reverse Heart Disease: The Revolutionary, Scientifically Proven, Nutrition-Based Cure.* 2007, Avery: Amazon.

18. Gilman, S. and T.V.d. Lestrade, *The Science of Fasting (Documentary).* 2015, YouTube: https://www.youtube.com/watch?v=t1bo8X-GvRs.

19. SS&M_Trustees *The Future of Social Security & Medicare (SS&M).* https://www.pgpf.org/blog/2019/04/five-charts-about-the-future-of-social-security-and-medicare, 2019. **Trustees Social Security & Medicare**

20. Benjamin, E., et al., *Heart Disease and Stroke Statistics: 2018 Update*, in *American Heart Association Report.* 2018, American Heart Association: American Heart Association Report. p. e67-e492.

21. ADA, *Economic Costs of Diabetes in the U.S. in 2017.* American Diabetes Association, 2017. **218;41(5)**(Diabetes Care): p. 917-928.

22. Finkelstein, E., et al., *Annual Medical Spending Attributable to Obesity: Payer and service-specific estimates.* Health Affairs., 2009. **(Millwood) Sep-Oct 2009;28(5)**(10.1377): p. w822-W831.

23. CDC, *The Cost of Arthritis in U.S. Adults.* Centers for Disease Control and Prevention, 2013.

24. Fung, J., *The Obesity Code: Unlocking the secrets of weight loss.* 1st ed. 2016, Vancouver, Canada: Greystone Books.

25. Zimmerman, M. *Why Some Communities of Color Have Been Hit so Much Harder by COVID-19: Pandemic amplifies the ethnic and socioeconomic gaps in health care.* AARP

    https://www.aarp.org/health/conditions-treatments/info-2020/race-coronavirus-disparities.html, 2020.

26. Marmot, M., et al., *Closing the Gap in a Generation: Health Equity through Action on the Social Determinants of Health.* Lancet, 2008. **372**(9650): p. 1661-1669.

27. Bowen-Matthew, D., *Just Medicine: A Cure for Racial Inequality in American Health Care.* 2015, New York University Press. p. 287.

28. Rosling, H., *Factfullness.* 2020, Amazon.

29. Lustig, R.H., *What is Metabolic Syndrome? Anyway (Lecture)* 2019, YouTube: https://www.youtube.com/watch?v=zx-QrilOoSM.

30. Hawkins, M. *10 Reasons Obamacare Is a Failure.* ThoughtCo

    https://www.thoughtco.com/reasons-obamacare-is-and-will-continue-to-be-a-failure-3303662, 2019, June 21.

31. Emanuel, E.J. *Why I Hope to Die at 75.* https://www.theatlantic.com/magazine/archive/2014/10/why-i-hope-to-die-at-75/379329/, 2014, October. **The Atlantic**

32. Taubes, G., *Good Calories, Bad Calories: Challenging the Conventional Wisdom on Diet, Weight Control, and Disease.* 2007, Alfred A. Knopf: Amazon.

33. Merriam-Webster, *Medical Words Definition*, in *Merriam-Webster Medical Dictionary*. 2020, Merriam-Webster.

34. Fung, J., *How Calories Are All Different*, in YouTube, Editor. 2020, YouTube: https://www.youtube.com/watch?v=_nt6KAUvedI.

35. deCabo, R. and M.P. Mattson, *Effects of Intermittent Fasting on Health, Aging, and Disease*. The New England Journal of Medicine, 2019(DOI: 10.1056/NEJMra1905136).

36. Patterson, R.E., et al., *Intermittent Fasting and Human Metabolic Health*. Journal of the Academy of Nutrition and Dietetics, 2016. **1203–12. doi:10.1016/j.jand.2015.02.018**: p. 115.

37. Fung, J., *The Diabetes Code: Prevent and Reverse Type 2 Diabetes Naturally*. 2018, Greystone Books: Amazon.

38. AHA_News *Time-restricted eating is growing in popularity, but is it healthy?* American Heart Association, 2019, Mar. 22.

39. Hatori, M., et al. *Time-Restricted Feeding without Reducing Caloric Intake Prevents Metabolic Diseases in Mice Fed a High-Fat Diet*. https://www.sciencedirect.com/science/article/pii/S1550413112001891, 2012. **Vol. 15**, 848-860.

40. Fung, J., *The Cancer Code: A Revolutionary New Understanding of a Medical Mystery*. 2020: Amazon.

41. What_I've_learned, *Why are people so Healthy in Japan?* In *https://www.youtube.com/watch?v=4WiUQtOhfIc*. 2018, YouTube: What_I've_learned.

42. Southside_Tokyo_News, *Western Diet: A killer in Okinawa*. 2009, YouTube: https://www.youtube.com/watch?v=8teAABsnTmM.

43. Hooper, R., *Obesity on the rise as Japanese eat more Western-style food*, in *The Japan Times*. 2012, Mar. 11: Tokyo, Japan.

44. Narayanan, A. *Western diet tied to heart risks in Asia*. ABC News in Science, 2012, July 23.

45. Odegaard, A.O., et al., *Western-Style Fast Food Intake and Cardiometabolic Risk in an Eastern Country*. Circulation, 2012. **126 No. 2**.

46. Taubes, G. *Is Sugar Toxic?* https://www.nytimes.com/2011/04/17/magazine/mag-17Sugar-t.html, 2011, April 17.

47. Lustig, R.H., *Is a Calorie a Calorie? Processed Food, Experiment Gone Wrong (Lecture)* 2015, YouTube: https://www.youtube.com/watch?v=nxyxcTZccsE.

48. O'Connor, A. *Why Eating Processed Foods Might Make You Fat.* https://www.nytimes.com/2019/05/16/well/eat/why-eating-processed-foods-might-make-you-fat.html, 2019, Mar. 16.

49. Open_Food_Facts *Nova Groups for Food Processing.* https://world.openfoodfacts.org/nova, 2019. **OpenFoodFacts.org**.

50. Lustig, R., *What Ultra-Processed Foods Do to Your Body*. 2019, YouTube: https://www.youtube.com/watch?v=_3UUR6FWCPA.

51. Bittman, M. and D. Katz, *How to Eat: All Your Food and Diet Questions Answered.* 2020, Houghton Mifflin Harcourt: Amazon

52. Schlosser, E.M., *Fast Food Nation: The Dark Side of the All-American Meal.* 2002, Houghton Mifflin Harcourt Publishing.

53. Bateman-House, A., et al., *Free to Consume? Anti-Paternalism and the Politics of New York City's Soda Cap Saga* Oxford Academy, Public Health Ethics 2017. **Volume 11**(Issue 1): p. Pages 45–53.

54. Lustig, R.H., *Sugar Has 56 Names: A Shopper's Guide*. 2013, Avery: Amazon. p. 184.

55. Oxner, R. *For Subway, A Ruling Not So Sweet. Irish Court Says Its Bread Isn't Bread..* https://www.npr.org/2020/10/01/919189045/for-subway-a-ruling-not-so-sweet-irish-court-says-its-bread-isnt-bread, 2020, Oct. 20.

56. Feehley, T. and C.R. Nagler, *The Weighty Costs of Non-Caloric Sweeteners.* Nature, 2014. **514**: p. 176-177.

57. AHA_Staff *How much sugar is too much?* Heart Attack and Stroke Symptoms, 2019.

58. Finca_Varsovia, *How we Craft our Finest Sugar - Panela - From Raw Sugarcane-Finca Varsovia Colombia*. 2018, YouTube: https://www.youtube.com/watch?v=cS6QVP2BBqw.

59. Rings_Gaston, *Process of Making Panela (Unrefined Sugar Cane), Trapiche (Process) in a Colombia Farm*, in *https://www.youtube.com/watch?v=1K6XKadWWq8*. 2014, YouTube.

60. Shanahan, C., *Deep Nutrition: Why Your Genes Need Traditional Food.* 2017, Flatiron books: Amazon.

61. Wright, B. *Heart-Healthy Fats: 5 Steps to Balance Omega Fatty Acids.* https://chopra.com/articles/heart-healthy-fats-5-steps-to-balance-omega-fatty-acids, 2017.

62. Knobbe, C., *'Diseases of Civilization: Are Seed Oil Excesses the Unifying Mechanism?* 2020, YouTube: https://www.youtube.com/watch?v=7kGnfXXIKZM.

63. Chris A Knobbe, *Ancestral Dietary Strategy to Prevent & Treat Macular Degeneration.* 2019, 2nd ed. Cure AMD Foundation: Amazon.

64. Fahy, E., et al., *Update of the LIPID MAPS comprehensive classification system for lipids.* Journal of Lipid Research, 2009. **50: S9-S14**: p. S9-S14.

65. Spiteller, D. and G. Spiteller, *Oxidation of Linoleic Acid in Low-Density Lipoprotein: An Important Event in Atherogenesis.* Angewandte Chemie International Edition, 2000. **39 (3)**: p. 585-589.

66. Vega-López, S., et al., *Palm and partially hydrogenated soybean oils adversely alter lipoprotein profiles compared with soybean and canola oils in moderately hyperlipidemic subjects* The American Journal of Clinical Nutrition, 2006. **84, July 2006**(1): p. 54-62.

67. Ekberg, S., *Top 10 Cooking Oils ... The Good, Bad, and Toxic.* 2021, YouTube: https://www.youtube.com/watch?v=pljQrjiDC9Q.

68. Taubes, G., *The Soft Science of Dietary Fat.* Science, 2001, Mar. 30. **291**(5513): p. 2536-2545.

69. Smith, A., *The Wealth of Nations*. 2016 (original publication 1776), Simon and Brown De Marque, Amazon.

70. Orwell, G., *Nineteen Eighty-Four*. 1st ed. 1949, New York: Harcourt, Brace and Company.

71. Linkins, J. *How Pizza Became A Vegetable Through The Magic Of Influence-Peddling*.. https://www.huffpost.com/entry/pizza-vegetable-school-lunches-lobbyists_n_1098029?, 2017, Dec 6.

72. Lustig, R.H., *The Hacking of the American Mind: The Science Behind the Corporate Takeover of Our Bodies and Brains*. 2017, Avery. p. 352.

73. Maturana, H.R. and B. Pörksen, *From Being to Doing: The Origins of the Biology of Cognition*. 2004, Carl-Auer Verlag. p. 246.

74. Senge, P.M., *The Fifth Discipline: The Art & Practice of The Learning Organization*. 2010, Currency. p. 466.

75. Shanahan, C., *How Vegetable Oils Lead To Insulin Resistance*, https://www.youtube.com/watch?v=_3_swYL6y_U, Editor. 2020, YouTube: YouTube.

76. Wechsler, M., *Sustainable (Documentary)*. 2017, YouTube: https://www.youtube.com/watch?v=xJuky56w7vI.

77. Open-Collab. *Purdue Pharma L.P. to Close the Company and Pay $8 Billion in Wikipedia*. Accessed 05/12/2021.

78. Maltus, T.R., *An Essay on the Principle of Population*. 1798, Amazon.

79. Khazan, O. *Why Are So Many Americans Dying Young?* https://www.theatlantic.com/health/archive/2016/12/why-are-so-many-americans-dying-young/510455/, 2016.

80. Daily_Chart *Why are Americans' lives getting shorter? A new analysis of life expectancy in the world's richest large country paints a bleak picture*. https://www.economist.com/graphic-detail/2019/11/27/why-are-americans-lives-getting-shorter, 2019.

81. Blaha, M.J. *5 Vaping Facts You Need to Know*. https://www.hopkinsmedicine.org/health/wellness-and-prevention/5-truths-you-need-to-know-about-vaping, 2020.

82. U.S.FDA *Final Determination Regarding Partially Hydrogenated Oils (Removing Trans Fat).* https://www.fda.gov/food/food-additives-petitions/final-determination-regarding-partially-hydrogenated-oils-removing-trans-fat, 2015. **Generally Recognized as Safe (GRAS)**.

83. Boesen, U. *Cigarette Taxes and Cigarette Smuggling by State, 2018*. Tax Foundation, 2020.

84. Senge, P., *Systems Thinking for a Better World (Lecture)*. 2020, YouTube: https://www.youtube.com/watch?v=0QtQqZ6Q5-0.

85. Braidwood, R.J., *Prehistoric Men*. 2016, Chicago Natural History Museum Press: Amazon.

86. Harari, Y.N., *Sapiens: A Brief History of Humankind*. 2015, HarperCollins Publishers: Amazon.

87. Plant_Based_News, *Lentils: A Miracle of Nutrition (Documentary)*, in *The United Kingdom*. 2019, YouTube: https://www.youtube.com/watch?v=1zzA9XA67ew.

88. Taubes, G., *The Qualities of Calories: lessons from the front line, Zurich & LCHF in practice.*, in *https://www.youtube.com/watch?v=5hGyKbsQCuk*. 2019, YouTube.

89. Segal, E. and E. Elinav, *The Personalized Diet: The Pioneering Program to Lose Weight and Prevent Disease*. 2017, Hachette Book Group: Amazon.

90. Zeevi, D., et al., *Personalized nutrition by prediction of glycemic responses*. Cell, 2015. **Cell 163, 1079–1094**.

91. Segal, E., *What is the best diet for humans?* 2016, YouTube: https://www.youtube.com/watch?v=0z03xkwFbw4.

92. Wahls, T. and E. Adamson, *The Wahls Protocol: A Radical New Way to Treat All Chronic Autoimmune Conditions Using Paleo Principles*. 2020, Avery: Amazon.

93. Ornish, D., *Dr. Dean Ornish's Program for Reversing Heart Disease: The Only System Scientifically Proven to Reverse Heart Disease Without Drugs or Surgery*. 1995, Ivy Books: Amazon.

94. Westman, E.C., S.D. Phinney, and J.S. Volek, *The New Atkins for a New You: The Ultimate Diet for Shedding Weight and Feeling Great*. 2010, Atria Books: Amazon.

95. Fung, J., *Fasting as a Therapeutic Option for Weight Loss (Lecture)*. 2019, YouTube: https://www.youtube.com/watch?v=7nJgHBbEgsE.

96. Armstrong, K., *The Great Transformation: The Beginning of Our Religious Traditions*. 2006, Anchor Books. p. 592.

97. McDonald, R.L., *The Complete Hamburger: Beyond the Golden Arches*. 2016, MHG Publishing: Amazon.

98. Kroc, R., *Grinding It Out*. 2016, St. Martin's Paperbacks: Amazon.

99. Sinclair, U., *The Fasting Cure: Reset Your Body*. 1911, Spruce and Alder Books: Amazon.

100. Fung, J. and J. Moore, *The Complete Guide to Fasting: Heal Your Body Through Intermittent, Alternate-Day, and Extended Fasting*. 2016, Victory Belt Publishing. p. 304.

101. deCabo, R. and M.P. Mattson, *Effects of Intermittent Fasting on Health, Aging, and Disease*. New England Journal of Medicine, 2019. **381**: p. 2541-2551.

102. Whitehead, M., G. Dahlgren, and T. Evans, *Equity and health sector reforms: Can low-income countries escape the medical poverty trap?* Lancet, 2001. **358 (9284): 833-36**: p. 833-36.

103. FDA_Food_Safety, *Arsenic in Rice and Rice Products Risk Assessment Report*, C.f.F.S.a.A. Nutrition, Editor. 2016, FDA: https://www.fda.gov/files/food/published/Arsenic-in-Rice-and-Rice-Products-Risk-Assessment-Report-PDF.pdf.

104. FDA, U.S. *What We Do*. https://www.fda.gov/about-fda/what-we-do, 2020.

105. Williams, B. *Side Effects Of Food Additives And Chemicals*. FIT, 2020.

106. Julia, C., F. Etile, and S. Hercberg, *Front-of-pack Nutri-Score labelling in France: an evidence-based policy*. The Lancet, 2018.

107. Global_Health_Metrics, *Global, regional, and national comparative risk assessment*

of 84 behavioural, environmental and occupational, and

metabolic risks or clusters of risks, 1990–2016: a systematic

analysis for the Global Burden of Disease Study 2016. The Lancet, 2017. **390 - Global Health Metrics.**

108. Monteiro, C.A., et al., *The UN Decade of Nutrition, the NOVA food classification and the trouble with ultra-processing*. Public Health Nutrition - Cambridge University, 2017. **21**(Special Issue 1): p. 5-17.

109. Fotsis, T., et al., *Genistein, a dietary-derived inhibitor of in vitro angiogenesis*. Proceedings of the National Academy of Sciences, 1993. **90**(7): p. 2690-2694.

110. Li, W.W., *Eat to Beat Disease: The New Science of How Your Body Can Heal Itself*. 2019, Grand Central Publishing. p. 414.

111. Lustig, R.H., et al., *Isocaloric fructose restriction and metabolic improvement in children with obesity and metabolic syndrome*. Pediatric Obesity, 2015. **24**(2).

112. Brownell, K.D., *Food Fight: The Inside Story of America's Obesity Crisis - and What We Can Do About It* 2003, McGraw Hill Education: Amazon.

113. Longo, V., *The Longevity Diet: Discover the New Science Behind Stem Cell Activation and Regeneration to Slow Aging, Fight Disease, and Optimize Weight*. 2018.

114. Credit_Suisse_Research_Institute *Sugar: Consumption at a Crossroad*. Credit Suisse Research Institute, 2013, September.

115. Mariotto, A., et al., *Cancer Prevalence and Cost of Care Projections: 2010-2020*. Journal National Cancer Institute, 2011. **103(2):117–128.**

116. Kotkin, J., *The Next Hundred Million: America in 2050*. 2010, The Penguin Press: Amazon.

117. Peter_G._Peterson_Foundation *Five charts about the future of Social Security and Medicare*. Peter_G._Peterson_Foundation

2019, April 23.

118. Open-Collab. *Cuba; Special Period. In Wikipedia.* https://en.wikipedia.org/wiki/Special_Period, Accessed 06/14/2020

119. Guerra, R., *Historia de Cuba I.* 2020, Linkgua: Amazon.

120. Sears, K., *U.S. History 101: Historic Events, Key People, Important Locations, and More!* 2014, Adams Media: Amazon-Simon & Schuster ebook.

121. Captivating_History, *History of Havana: A Captivating Guide to the History of the Capital of Cuba, Starting from Christopher Columbus' Arrival to Fidel Castro.* 2018, Captivating History: Amazon.

122. Captivating_History, *History of Cuba: A Captivating Guide to Cuban History, Starting from Christopher Columbus' Arrival to Fidel Castro.* 2018, Captivating History: Amazon.

123. Guerra, R., *Historia de Cuba II.* 2019, Linkgua: Amazon.

124. Lopez, A.J., *José Martí: A Revolutionary Life.* 2014, University of Texas Press: Amazon.

125. Hourly_History, *Spanish American War: A History From Beginning to End.* 2016, Hourly History: Amazon.

126. Thomas, H., *Cuba: La lucha por la libertad (Spanish Edition),* in *La lucha por la libertad.* 2002: Amazon.

127. Captivating_History, *The Cuban Revolution: A Captivating Guide to the Armed Revolt That Changed the Course of Cuba, Including Stories of Leaders Such as Fidel Castro, Chè Guevara, and Fulgencio Batista* C. History, Editor. 2018, Captivating History: Amazon.

128. Open-Collab. *United States Embargo Against Cuba. In Wikipedia.* https://en.wikipedia.org/wiki/United_States_embargo_against_Cuba, Accessed 07/18/2020.

129. Hourly_History, *The Cuban Missile Crisis: A History From Beginning to End.* 2018, Hourly History: Amazon.

130. Open-Collab. *José Martí Pioneer Organization in Wikipedia.* https://en.wikipedia.org/wiki/Jos%C3%A9_Mart%C3%AD_Pioneer_Organization, 2019.

131. Werlau, M.C., *La intervención de Cuba en Venezuela: Una ocupación estratégica con implicaciones globales (Spanish Edition)* in *Una ocupación estratégica con implicaciones globales* 2019: Amazon.

132. Larzelere, A., *Castro's Ploy: America's Dilemma: The 1980 Cuban Boatlift*, in *The 1980 Cuban Boatlift*

2020: Amazon.

133. Pérez-López, J. *The Cuban Economic Crisis of the 1990s and the External Sector.* The Association for the Study of the Cuban Economy (ASCE)

https://www.ascecuba.org/asce_proceedings/the-cuban-economic-crisis-of-the-1990s-and-the-external-sector/, 1998, Nov. 30.

134. Plinio-Montalvan, G. *Cuba 1990–1994: Political Intransigence versus Economic Reform.* ASCE, 1994.

135. Warner, R. *Is the Cuban healthcare system really as great as people claim?* The Conversation

https://theconversation.com/is-the-cuban-healthcare-system-really-as-great-as-people-claim-69526, 2016.

136. Lamrani, S., *Cuba's Health Care System: A Model for the World.* 2014, Opera Mundi: Sao Paolo.

137. Whiteford, L.M. and L.G. Branch, *Primary Health Care in Cuba: The Other Revolution.* 2007, Rowman & Littlefield: Amazon.

138. Nordlinger, J. *The Myth of Cuban Health Care.* National Review

https://www.nationalreview.com/2007/07/myth-cuban-health-care/, 2007, July 11.

139. Orwell, G., *Animal Farm.* 1945, Secker and Warburg: Amazon.

140. Panichelli-Batalla, S. *Castro's legacy: Cuban doctors still go abroad, but it's no longer driven by international solidarity.* The Conversation

https://theconversation.com/castros-legacy-cuban-doctors-still-go-abroad-but-its-no-longer-driven-by-international-solidarity-65181, 2016, Nov. 30.

141. Cuban_Institute_of_Ophthalmology *Cuban Health Services.* https://www.cubamundomedico.com/en/cuban-institute-of-ophthalmology, 2019.

142. 14ymedio *Cuba's Doctors of the Miracle Mission are Simple "Catarologists, (Technicians)" Reveals Uruguay Newspaper*

http://translatingcuba.com/cubas-doctors-of-the-miracle-mission-are-simple-catarologists-reveals-uruguay-newspaper/, 2019, Dec. 9.

143. Cuba-History *Special Period and Recovery.* https://www.cubahistory.org/en/special-period-a-recovery.html, 1999.

144. Vogel, E.F., *Deng Xiaoping and the Transformation of China.* 2011: Amazon.

145. Top10, *Top 20 Economies 2021 (Nominal GDP).* 2021, YouTube: https://www.youtube.com/watch?v=iiJDdmx7R_A.

146. Norberg, J., *The Real Adam Smith: Ideas That Changed The World*, in *https://www.youtube.com/watch?v=8ruiUOQERnw*. 2016, YouTube: YouTube.

147. Luis, L.R. *Cuba Restructures Its Visible External Debt.* https://www.ascecuba.org/cuba-restructures-visible-external-debt/, 2016, Jan. 10.

148. Fung, J., *The Roots of the Obesity Epidemic (Lecture).* 2019, YouTube: https://www.youtube.com/watch?v=q8BGYhreaco.

149. Open-Collab. *Food Rationing in Cuba. In Wikipedia.* https://en.wikipedia.org/wiki/Rationing_in_Cuba, Accessed 04/06/2020.

150. Weiner, R., *The New York City Soda Ban Explained*, in *The Washington Post*. 2013, March 11, The Washington Post:

https://www.washingtonpost.com/news/the-fix/wp/2013/03/11/the-new-york-city-soda-ban-explained/.

151. ISO_Internet *International Sugar Organization Our Role.* https://www.isosugar.org/aboutus/role-of-the-international-sugar-organization, Accessed 12/28/2020.

152. Banting, W., *The Banting Diet: Letter on Corpulence.* 2015, Cosimo Classics (original work published 1864): Amazon.

153. Burke, B. *Shipyards, a Crucible for Tragedy Part 1: How the war created a monster.* https://www.asbestos-attorney.com/pilot3-1.htm, 2001, May 6.

154. Open-Collab. *Lead Paint. In Wikipedia.* https://en.wikipedia.org/wiki/Lead_paint, Accessed 09/21/2020.

155. Kovarik, W. *Milestones: Leaded gasoline: How a Classic Occupational Disease Became an International Public Health Disaster.* INTERNATIONAL JOURNAL OCCUPATIONAL ENVIRONMENTAL HEALTH 2005. **VOL 11/NO 4**.

156. Doll, R. and A.B. Hill, *Smoking and carcinoma of the lung*. British Medical Journal, 1950. **2:739**(2:739).

157. Mayo_Clinic_Staff *Trans fat is double trouble for your heart health.* https://www.mayoclinic.org/diseases-conditions/high-blood-cholesterol/in-depth/trans-fat/art-20046114, 2020.

158. Merriam-Webster *Metabolism. In Merriam-Webster.com.* https://unabridged.merriam-webster.com/medical/metabolism, 2020, Aug. 10.

159. Lustig, R.H., *Frontiers of Science (Lecture).* 2014, YouTube: https://www.youtube.com/watch?v=uIIXUZwpB-U.

160. Lustig, R.H., *Sugar: The Bitter Truth (Lecture).* 2009, YouTube: https://www.youtube.com/watch?v=dBnniua6-oM.

161. Fung, J., *The Aetiology of Obesity.* 2016, YouTube: https://www.youtube.com/watch?v=ZKC3hiyLeRc.

162. Ohsumi, Y. *Autophagy: The Nobel Prize in Physiology or Medicine 2016.* https://www.nobelprize.org/prizes/medicine/2016/press-release/, 2016, Oct. 30.

163. Bauer, R.A., E. Collar, and V. Tang, *The Silverlake Project: Transformation at IBM*. 1992: Oxford University Press. 240.

****

INDEX

The page numbers in this index refer to the printed version of this book. You may need to use the e-reader search tool for the digital edition to find the appropriate reference location or page.

A

B

C

D

E

F

G

H

I

J

K

L

M

N

O

P

S

T

U

V

W

* * * * * * * * * * * * * * *

www.ingramcontent.com/pod-product-compliance
Lightning Source LLC
Chambersburg PA
CBHW050109280326
41933CB00010B/1023

* 9 7 8 0 5 7 8 8 4 9 5 3 9 *